COGNITIVE BEHAVIOURAL THERAPY FOR CHILD TRAUMA AND ABUSE

of related interest

Cool Connections with Cognitive Behavioural Therapy
Encouraging Self-Esteem, Resilience and Wellbeing in Children and Young People Using CBT Approaches
Laurie Seiler
ISBN 978 1 84310 618 0

Breaking Free from OCD
A CBT Guide for Young People and Their Families
Jo Derisley, Isobel Heyman, Sarah Robinson and Cynthia Turner
Illustrated by Lisa Jo Robinson
ISBN 978 1 84310 574 9

Therapy to Go
Gourmet Fast Food Handouts for Working with Child, Adolescent and Family Clients
Clare Rosoman
ISBN 978 1 84310 643 2

Children and Adolescents in Trauma
Creative Therapeutic Approaches
Edited by Chris Nicholson, Michael Irwin and Kedar N. Dwivedi
Foreword by Peter Wilson
ISBN 978 1 84310 437 7
Community, Culture and Change Series

Safeguarding Children Living with Trauma and Family Violence
Evidence-Based Assessment, Analysis and Planning Interventions
Arnon Bentovim, Anthony Cox, Liz Bingley Miller and Stephen Pizzey
Foreword by Brigid Daniel
ISBN 978 1 84310 938 9
Best Practice in Working with Children Series

Mental Health Interventions and Services for Vulnerable Children and Young People
Edited by Panos Vostanis
Foreword by Richard Williams
ISBN 978 1 84310 489 6

Creative Coping Skills for Children
Emotional Support through Arts and Crafts Activities
Bonnie Thomas
ISBN 978 1 84310 921 1

Introduction to Counselling Survivors in Interpersonal Trauma
Christiane Sanderson
ISBN 978 1 84310 962 4

COGNITIVE BEHAVIOURAL THERAPY FOR CHILD TRAUMA AND ABUSE
A STEP-BY-STEP APPROACH

Jacqueline S. Feather and Kevin R. Ronan

Illustrated by Duncan Innes

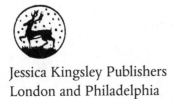

Jessica Kingsley Publishers
London and Philadelphia

First published in 2010
by Jessica Kingsley Publishers
116 Pentonville Road
London N1 9JB, UK
and
400 Market Street, Suite 400
Philadelphia, PA 19106, USA

www.jkp.com

Library of Congress Cataloging in Publication Data
Feather, Jacqueline S., 1954-
  Cognitive behavioural therapy for child trauma and abuse : a step-by-step approach /
Jacqueline S. Feather and Kevin R. Ronan ; illustrated by Duncan Innes.
    p. ; cm.
  Includes bibliographical references.
  ISBN 978-1-84905-086-9 (alk. paper)
  1. Cognitive therapy for children. 2. Psychic trauma in children--Treatment. I. Ronan, Kevin R. II. Title.
  [DNLM: 1. Cognitive Therapy--methods. 2. Adolescent. 3. Child Abuse--therapy.
  4. Child. 5. Stress Disorders, Post-Traumatic--therapy. WS 350.6 F288c 2010]
  RJ505.C63F43 2010
  618.92'89142--dc22

                    2009049839

British Library Cataloguing in Publication Data
A CIP catalogue record for this book is available from the British Library

ISBN 978 1 84905 086 9

Printed and bound in Great Britain by
MPG Books Group

Contents

ACKNOWLEDGEMENTS

It is with pleasure and gratitude that we acknowledge all those who have been instrumental in bringing this book into reality. We also wish to acknowledge clinicians who work with traumatised and abused children, and hope that this book will contribute to your work with this most vulnerable population.

We especially acknowledge the work of the team of therapists and researchers, including Kevin R. Ronan, at the Child and Adolescent Anxiety Disorders Clinic at Temple University, who originally developed and trialled the cognitive behavioural programme that inspired this intervention programme and this book. In addition, we would like to acknowledge Liana Lowenstein for her interventions for troubled youth that she has kindly allowed us to incorporate into our programme (Lowenstein 2000). Leah Giarratano for permission to use the TRAP model (Giarratano 2004); and Christine Padesky for her gracious permission in allowing us to reprint and adapt for children the 5-part model diagram (Greenberg and Padesky 1995, p.4). We also wish to thank Associate Professor Paul Merrick, of Massey University, for his synopsis of the essential elements of CBT (Merrick 1999), and for his valuable guidance and editorial support.

The development and initial evaluation of this treatment model was made possible in part by a doctoral scholarship granted to Jacqueline S. Feather by Massey University, and a grant-in-aid by the New Zealand Government's Ministry of Social Policy.

We specifically acknowledge the excellent work and support of the therapists and staff at the Specialist Services Unit (SSU) of the Department of Child, Youth and Family, Auckland, New Zealand, who aided in the development and evaluation of this programme.

In particular, we would like to acknowledge the contributions made by the following people, who provided consultation, advice, research assistance and support: Tina Berking, Dr Nici Curtis, Dr Mary Dawson, Ngaire Eruera, Robyn Girling-Butcher, Sue Hutchinson, Dr Caryl Huzziff, Dr Heather McDowell, Frances Miller, Paora Murupaenga, Angela Person, Yvonne Pink, Virginia Tamanui, Jonathan Tolcher, Caryn Trent, Sunila Wilson, Caroline Witten-Hannah, Louise Woolf; and in Australia, Marcella Cline, Kaylene Paradine, and the therapists at Wahroonga Counselling Centre, Rockhampton, Australia.

For the illustrations, special acknowledgement to Duncan Innes who took the time to listen to what we wanted, and then put his own creative spin on the images to produce ideas beyond our expectations.

To the publishers, Jessica Kingsley Publishers, and, in particular, to our editors, Stephen Jones and Claire Cooper, thank you for your patience, helpful suggestions and belief in this work.

Last, but not least, a very big thank you to the children and families who participated in the research underpinning the development of this therapy programme, and to family and friends who provided endless encouragement and practical and emotional support; in particular, Jackie's husband Tim, adult children Nicola, Ben and Gabrielle, and their partners; and Kevin's wife Isabel and two gorgeous daughters, Emily and Kaitlin.

INTRODUCTION

This book describes a trauma-focused cognitive behavioural therapy (TF-CBT) programme for children and young adolescents (aged 9–15 years) who have posttraumatic stress disorder (PTSD) symptoms as the result of child abuse and related traumatic experiences. The step-by-step approach is presented in a 16-session format designed to be adapted for each individual child. Four sessions for parents/caregivers are included, one at the beginning of each 'phase' of the programme.

Research and development

The model was originally developed by clinicians in a real-world setting for treating multiply abused and traumatised children (Feather and Ronan 2004). It was based on (1) a review of the child abuse and trauma literature, with particular reference to professional developments and the role of psychologists and therapists in ameliorating the effects; (2) a conceptualisation of the clinical presentation of child abuse and trauma in children; (3) a review of the field of psychotraumatology and relevant theoretical models; (4) a review of evidence-based practice, treatment outcome models, and current empirical research related to developing an effective treatment model in this area (Feather 2008). Essentially, this TF-CBT programme built on local practice and empirically supported treatments for child anxiety (Kendall *et al.* 1992; Kendall, Kane, Howard and Siqueland 1989) and PTSD as the result of sexual abuse (e.g., Deblinger and Heflin 1996). It has been evaluated in a series of single-case design treatment outcome studies, with promising results (Feather and Ronan 2006, 2009b; Feather *et al.* n.d.).

Empirical evidence is strongest for cognitive-behavioural approaches over other forms of psychotherapy for efficacy in resolving PTSD and other anxiety-related symptoms in children (Cohen, Berliner and March 2000; Compton *et al.* 2002), and TF-CBT is recommended for treating the specific problems of abused children (Saunders, Berliner, and Hanson 2001). Support has been found for the efficacy of the TF-CBT approach in treating a range of traumatic experiences (Cohen *et al.* 2004; Deblinger, Stauffer and Steer 2001; King *et al.* 2000; March *et al.* 1998). This treatment approach incorporates psychoeducation, coping skills training via behavioural interventions such as emotional expression and relaxation, and cognitive interventions such as coping self-talk and problem-solving. Gradual exposure techniques are utilised for trauma processing. The intervention is delivered primarily as individual therapy, with sessions for parents/caregivers to provide psychoeducation and support and enable the transfer of what is learned in therapy to the child's[1] home environment.

The 16-session step-by-step format was inspired by, and is adapted from, a 16-session manualised CBT intervention for the treatment of anxiety disorders in children and young adolescents developed by a team that included the second author (Kendall *et al.* 1992; Kendall *et al.* 1989; Ronan and Deane 1998). This intervention model focuses on the acquisition and practice of coping skills to help the child manage anxiety symptoms.

A key consideration in adapting an anxiety-based approach to the treatment of PTSD symptoms was that anxiety is about current and future threat whereas PTSD, while an anxiety disorder, has much to do with past event(s). Children who have PTSD symptoms are processing trauma and/or its sequelae in a way that involves ongoing distress (Ehlers and Clark 2000). Hence, in adapting elements from the original anxiety management programme, the aim of the current TF-CBT intervention was to include a number of additional elements specific to treating ongoing trauma and abuse related sequelae, to help children develop skills to manage their symptoms, and to process their traumatic experience so that it is seen as time-limited past event(s) that can be managed effectively by the child and his[2] family/caregivers.

A second major consideration in the development of this treatment programme has been the psychosocial context of traumatised children. Traumatic experiences often affect the relationships children have with their parents, family members, peers and others. It may mean the involvement of other adults in their lives, such as police, social workers and other helping professionals. In the case of child abuse, children may be placed in temporary or permanent care to ensure their safety. Removal from parents not only adds another layer to the trauma for these young people, but also necessitates forming new relationships with caregivers. The early part of the treatment is devoted to exploring and strengthening the child's psychosocial context, as a basis for the later treatment interventions.

Clearly, a child's attachment experiences can impact on the development of the relationship with the therapist, and time spent by the therapist exploring and strengthening the child's psychosocial context can provide ample opportunities for rapport building. This programme is not designed specifically to address attachment issues, but it is anticipated that the facilitation of a positive therapeutic relationship will be helpful for children, some of whom may have had little experience of safe secure attachment relationships. There are also a number of other contextual factors that must be in place to enable the best possible outcome from TF-CBT for the child and family. These include child safety, parent/caregiver involvement, cultural considerations and tailoring treatment to the individual child's experiences and traumatic responses.

---

1   While this therapy is appropriate for young adolescents as well as children, the word 'child' will be used throughout the book to refer to the young client.

2   To increase readability and not intending any particular connotation, throughout the book the child will be referred to in the masculine and the therapist in the feminine.

Child safety and parent/caregiver involvement

For any child therapy to be effective, it is essential that the child is in a safe home environment and that there is support for the therapeutic process outside of the therapy room. The inclusion of parent/caregiver sessions enables the ongoing involvement of one or more significant safe adults in the treatment programme. These sessions are designed to give the adult(s) ongoing information about components of the programme and the child's progress, and to allow opportunity for their questions and feedback. The sessions include psychoeducation about the effects of traumatic experiences on children, demonstration of coping skills, encouragement to help the child to apply and practise these skills at home, and assistance in supporting the child throughout each stage of the programme. In addition, the therapist should liaise with the child's school and any other agencies involved, as necessary to support a successful outcome of therapy.

It is important to note that while this treatment programme involves parents and caregivers, it is not designed as an adult intervention *per se*. It is expected that any additional interventions that may be required by a child's offending or non-offending parent(s) will be provided alongside this programme by the appropriate services.

Underlying philosophy and principles

Just as a child cannot be fully understood without reference to his environment, it is important for clinicians implementing this treatment to be aware of the context in which this treatment programme was developed, and the principles that guide the approach. The step-by-step TF-CBT programme is essentially a tool for engagement and a kit of change-producing strategies. The cognitive behavioural model provides not only the techniques, but also the essential elements for change. Key among these, as already noted, is the therapeutic relationship. The nature of the relationship can have a powerful influence on therapy progress and outcomes. This TF-CBT programme is based on a particular view of the desirable elements of that relationship. It was developed in the unique context of Aotearoa[3]/New Zealand, which has as a founding document the Treaty of Waitangi – essentially an agreement for partnership between the indigenous Maori and the European settlers signed in 1840 by Maori chiefs and the British Crown. The Treaty continues to be a 'living document' that provides guidance for our bicultural nation.

The spirit of the principles of *partnership*, *participation* and *active protection* embodied in the Treaty of Waitangi strongly influence health policy and delivery (National Advisory Committee on Health and Disability 2002), and have been incorporated into this programme. To be explicit, *partnership* encourages working together in a spirit of co-operation; *participation* promotes active involvement of the child, family and caregivers; and *active protection* includes the idea of comprehensive monitoring to ensure improvement. These principles are nicely analogous to the essential elements of CBT, as described below.

Essentially, the TF-CBT programme[4] provides a model and means for partnership between the therapist and the child, his family and significant others, to enable acceptance and change.

---

3   *Aotearoa*: 'Land of the Long White Cloud'; the Maori name for New Zealand.

4   The Maori name for the programme, bestowed by Paora Murupaenga and used in New Zealand, is: *Te Ara Whetu*, 'the way lit by stars'.

Anyone who knows the New Zealand story will know that this is not always an easy process, but at best the bringing together of two cultures in a climate of respect and willingness to listen and learn from each other makes possible the creation of a new future which is acknowledging, enriching and rewarding for all.

In the case of the therapeutic relationship, it is the therapist who holds the responsibility for developing a partnership based on safety, respect, understanding and hope, which will give the child, with the support of his caregivers, the opportunity and possibility of creating a new future for himself. To facilitate this, the therapist should be aware of her own background and values and be emotionally available to the child in order to establish a therapeutic connection, with the wishes and needs of the child as paramount. The process of getting to know the child, his family, and something about his background and values provides the foundation for the therapeutic endeavour.

Cultural considerations

In the spirit of partnership, if the therapist and child are of different cultural or other type of backgrounds, it is expected that the therapist will respect difference and use cultural or other consultation. Consideration should be given to the child's and family's ethnic and cultural identity, as this is likely to influence the child's clinical presentation and response to treatment. For example, what feelings, thoughts and behaviours are facilitated and promoted as a function of the child's social or cultural context? Has the child and/or family experienced dislocation, encountered prejudice or marginalisation? How have these experiences shaped symptom expression? What beliefs about self, others and the world have been shaped by cultural and related experiences? Are there ongoing effects of racism, colonisation, migration or injustice? These experiences can obviously affect a child's progress in therapy. While this programme is not designed to address these factors directly, it is expected that the therapist will work collaboratively with the child and family to identify positive strategies for dealing with these kinds of adverse environmental situations, and to honour their heritage and cultural world view.

Within the therapy room itself, the therapist needs to be aware of how cultural and other individual differences can affect the therapeutic relationship. For example, different family and cultural groups may hold varying beliefs regarding obedience to authority; the way children and families relate to the therapist's 'authority' can influence their responses to therapy. Culture can shape linguistic and other courtesies and conventions, such as rhythm of speech, eye contact and rules for turn-taking in conversation; children will tell their stories in different ways. The therapist needs to adapt her rapport building and interventions accordingly. The programme is designed as a tool kit to be implemented within the child's and family's world view. It is in the clients' best interests that the therapist is culturally sensitive, respects their world view, and uses the CBT treatment strategies as appropriate within this context.

Research on the use of the TF-CBT programme with children and families of indigenous and migrant cultures in Aotearoa/New Zealand has confirmed the salience of a collaborative therapeutic relationship and the critical importance of interweaving models based on Western psychology with culturally different world views in order to facilitate best outcomes for clients (Feather 2008; Murupaenga, Feather and Berking 2004). In fact, with cultural supervision, one of us (JF) experienced a transition in thinking from a view that culture should be considered as part of a CBT approach, to a view that both should receive equal weighting, and a realisation that CBT is a tool for change that exists within cultural paradigms (P. Murupaenga, personal communication, 19 August 2004). The diagram below depicts this transition in thinking:

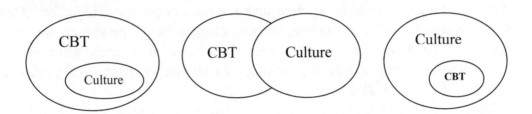

Overall, research and clinical experience in using TF-CBT with children and families of minority indigenous and migrant groups indicates that while CBT is not a cure-all to address wider issues of connection and identity, the TF-CBT programme is a useful tool in the context of a culturally sensitive, collaborative therapeutic relationship to facilitate healing from trauma and abuse-related symptoms and concerns.

Trauma and abuse-related presentations in children

Traumatic events may range from a single incident experienced by a child, such as an accident or natural disaster, to chronic abuse and neglect, and may in turn lead to a wide range of manifestations (Feather and Ronan 2009a). With regard to child abuse and interpersonal violence, research shows that many children who have had these experiences have been victimised on multiple occasions (Finkelhor *et al.* 2005). Of course, it should be kept in mind that, regardless of the nature of the experience, some children may demonstrate resilience, whereas others exhibit long-lasting effects. Traumatic sequelae in children may include emotional responses, bodily sensations, behavioural and cognitive responses. Terr found most cases of childhood trauma were characterised by: (1) trauma-specific fears, (2) strongly visualised or otherwise repeatedly perceived memories, (3) repetitive behaviours, and (4) changed attitudes about people, aspects of life and the future (Terr 1991). Terr distinguished between Type I trauma, resulting from one event, and Type II, resulting from long-standing or repeated ordeals. Relevant to this treatment programme is the important need to assess children with these distinctions in mind, as different presentations will require a different emphasis in treatment.

The diagnostic category of PTSD, while it does not specifically cover all the manifestations of more complex traumatic experiences, such as child abuse (Briere 1992; Herman 1992), is useful as a way of understanding children's experiences and determining targets for treatment. PTSD in children and adolescents is similar to PTSD in adults, including the cardinal symptoms of re-experiencing, avoidance/numbing and increased physiological arousal (Davis and Siegel 2000). The DSM-IV-TR (American Psychiatric Association 2000) describes the differential effects of trauma for children. For example, children may exhibit agitated or disorganised behaviour, nightmares about monsters or threats to self and others (not just specifically about the traumatic event itself), and may engage in repetitive acting out of the trauma. Chronic PTSD in maltreated children has been associated with helplessness, guilt, hyperarousal, avoidance, disturbances in memory and information processing, negative abuse related attributions and an avoidant coping style (Cohen and Mannarino 1996; Linning and Kearney 2004). Some children who are severely traumatised may not meet diagnostic criteria for PTSD, and may display symptoms such as disruptive, affective, dissociative and personality disordered features (Perry et al. 1995). Comorbid psychological disturbance, in particular other anxiety disorders and depression, as well as related problems, are common for traumatised and abused children (Linning and Kearney 2004).

There is considerable evidence to suggest that traumatic experiences as a child can have a profound effect on the developing brain (Nemeroff 2004). It has been proposed that complex traumas, such as may occur in the case of child abuse, can lead to overactivation of neural pathways (e.g., via experiencing a traumatic event), and/or deprivation of sensory stimuli (e.g., via disrupted attachment, neglect), which may in turn lead to a persistent pattern of hyperarousal or dissociation (Perry et al. 1995). In addition, many factors may influence the response to trauma (McFarlane and Yehuda 2000). The aetiology and course of PTSD and trauma-related effects in children is likely to be a complex function of developmental stage, prior experiences and temperament, parent and family functioning, subsequent coping, and reactions to secondary adversity (Pynoos 1994; Ronan and Johnson 2005). In fact, as we have stated elsewhere, a simplistic, linear view of PTSD (i.e., traumatic event = PTSD) will underestimate the complexity of trauma-related responses and lead to simplistic formulation and incomplete treatment plans (Feather and Ronan 2009a). A CBT approach can cater for the inherent complexity of working with trauma presentations, not least because it advocates for an ever-evolving formulation and a specific focus on the individual child's experience.

CBT essential elements

Essential elements of CBT[5] incorporated into this programme include the following.

- **The centrality of the cognitive behavioural conceptualisation.** The therapist develops an ever-evolving formulation of the child and his problems in cognitive behavioural terms – for example, by clarifying the life events, experiences and interactions that have led to and maintain the child's problems, and by ongoing assessment of the child's thoughts, feelings, behaviours and coping strategies.

- **The phenomenological emphasis.** The child's experience is the central focus of the therapy. The therapist 'sees the world through the child's eyes' and works with the child's view of himself, others and the world.

- **The collaborative nature of the therapeutic relationship.** The therapist's overall aim is to foster a relationship of equality and partnership with the child. This involves a collaborative 'team' approach whereby the child collects the raw data (in session work and homework tasks) to be investigated with the therapist's guidance. The skills required by the

---

5   Adapted from a lecture given by Paul Merrick (Merrick 1999).

therapist include genuineness, warmth and empathy, as well as the more specific skills of challenging and reinforcing the child's efforts at change in an open and direct but respectful way.

- **The active involvement of the child.** The child is actively involved in the therapy throughout – for example, in bringing situations to therapy to discuss via the homework tasks.

- **The use of Socratic questioning and guided discovery.** Rather than interpreting the child's thoughts and actions, the therapist uses open-ended questions (known as 'Socratic questioning') to help the child discover data for himself. Guided discovery includes empathic listening, frequent summarising, and asking synthesising and analytical questions.

- **Explicitness of the therapist.** The consistent therapy session structure allows for explicitness by means of frequent summaries and opportunities for feedback from the child. This allows the process of therapy to be more predictable for the child. In addition, the therapist regularly shares her ideas with the child about progress.

- **The emphasis on empiricism.** The therapist and child form hypotheses or ideas about what might help him manage his symptoms and feel better, and the child tests these in and out of the sessions, reviewing progress week by week.

- **The 'outward' focus.** The aim of CBT is to teach the child to become 'his own therapist'. The therapy is designed to facilitate the generalisation of in-session therapeutic change to everyday situations that he encounters. The outward focus is enhanced by the setting of out-of-session tasks, which is likely to lead to better outcomes and reduce relapse.

- **The importance of emotions.** The child is encouraged to identify and differentiate his feelings. He learns to rate the intensity of emotion to help identify problematic situations. Emotions are used to target interventions. For example, relaxation techniques are taught to help a child learn to calm down when upset; subjective rating scales are used to assess the effectiveness of interventions. The child is also helped to become aware of positive emotions and the links between thoughts, behaviours and situations which support him in feeling better.

- **The central role of exposure.** The therapist helps the child to face his fears and worries in a safe therapeutic environment, leading to a reduction in anxiety. Through learning and integrating new skills such as relaxation and changing his thoughts, the child is helped to respond differently to his symptoms and problems. Through gradual exposure the child learns that he can approach his fears without experiencing catastrophic consequences, leading to an overall reduction in avoidance behaviours in his everyday life.

- **The contextual framework.** The cognitive behavioural model considers a child's thoughts, feelings and behaviours not only in relation to specific situations but also in relation to his broader context. The therapist takes into account the finer nuances of antecedents and consequences of the child's presenting problems, as well as the interactive effects of his history and development, family relationships and attachments, and social and cultural context on his symptom expression and response to therapy.

Overview and rationale

The TF-CBT programme comprises four phases, presented within a 16-session format:

Phase One: Psychosocial Strengthening

Three sessions (Sessions 1–3) to provide an orientation to therapy, build rapport, elicit hope and active participation, gain information about the child's world and view of himself, explore family relationships and identify social supports; to begin to identify the child's history of trauma and current trauma symptoms, normalise reactions by providing psychoeducation about the effects of trauma on children, and introduce a coping model. Goals for therapy are established.

The rationale for this phase is to set the context for therapy. For example, some abused children have complex histories and social contexts which it is helpful for both therapist and child to begin to acknowledge and understand. This forms an important part of building the therapeutic relationship, and provides a basis for the therapy to follow.

In this phase any immediate concerns should be immediately addressed with behavioural interventions – for example, sleep problems with sleep hygiene, low mood with scheduling in positive activities, anxiety and emotional upsets with self-calming skills with quick relaxation interventions. Such efforts validate the child and anticipate the more comprehensive coping skills learned in the next phase.

Out-of-session 'self-help' tasks are introduced to help the child to begin to practise self-monitoring, and to create a bridge between therapy and his everyday life.

Phase Two: Coping Skills ('The STAR Plan')

Five sessions (Sessions 4–8) based on cognitive behavioural techniques which encourage children to cope directly with their anxiety and trauma symptoms, rather than relying on avoidance behaviours to reduce personal distress. The rationale for this phase of the treatment is that the strategies the child has used so far to deal with trauma memory may make sense, but may be maintaining the symptoms. The new coping strategies will help the child to know when he is upset and know what to do to feel better.

The coping skills are introduced to the child as a four-step 'coping template' for managing trauma symptoms, referred to as 'The STAR Plan'.[6] To assist the child to recall the four-step plan, the 'STAR' acronym and symbol is used:

- **S**cary feelings?
- **T**hinking bad things?
- **A**ctivities that can help
- **R**ating and rewards

---

6   Adapted from 'The FEAR Plan' (Kendall *et al.* 1989).

The first step involves training the child in recognition and management of feelings and body reactions, including those associated with anxiety and trauma. *The second step* assists the child to recognise thoughts, in particular his own 'self-talk', when he is upset. *The third step* involves modification of unhelpful self-talk into helpful self-talk and developing plans for coping more effectively with upsetting situations. *The fourth step* comprises self-rating and self-reward, even for partial success, to encourage the child to maintain his new skills and feel better.

The concepts and skills are introduced and practised in sequential order, from a focus on generalised and less stressful to more personal and more stressful situations. The therapist acts as a coping model, demonstrating and practising each new skill with the child. The child is invited to apply the ideas to imaginal situations through activities and role-plays. Finally, the child is encouraged to apply the concepts and skills to himself and his own situation.

Out-of-session self-monitoring ('self-help') tasks enable the child to apply and practise his newly acquired skills *in vivo*.

Phase Three: Trauma Processing (Gradual Exposure)

A series of sessions based on a cognitive behavioural model of how trauma symptoms are maintained. Any associations that continue to exist between anxiety and fear and the situations or thoughts which produce these sensations need to be processed. This is accomplished by gradually exposing the child to the upsetting situations until anxiety decreases (habituation). Coping skills are used to manage symptoms throughout the exposure phase. When habituation has occurred sufficiently, new associations can begin to replace old ones; that is, relaxed or non-anxious responses become connected to previously upsetting situations or thoughts. Gradual exposure in a safe therapeutic environment that prevents avoidance reinforces the child's learning that anxiety decreases without the need to use avoidance strategies. In addition, exposure techniques enable cognitive changes (Yule, Smith and Perrin 2005). When the child realises that facing a feared situation or thought does not result in threat and/or unabated anxiety, beliefs maintaining the trauma and anxiety may also change.

The therapist helps the child to remember and re-experience traumatic memories and the emotions engendered, in such a way that distress can be mastered rather than magnified. Using imaginal exposure techniques the child is asked to imagine and recount his traumatic experiences in the therapy room. Exposure is gradual in that the child chooses the least traumatic memories to work on first, gradually moving to the most traumatic. A range of modalities for imaginal exposure work are presented in the programme, including sand play, clay, art and puppets. The child chooses the modality he wishes to work with each session. The exposure sessions are paced to enable the child to feel in control and not experience overwhelming anxiety. At the same time, the therapist needs to ensure that the most difficult aspects of the traumatic experiences are examined in order for the exposure intervention to be successful.

The STAR Plan is used to help the child manage any symptoms that arise during exposure. The child is instructed in the use of SUDS (Subjective Units of Distress Scales) to rate his anxiety. The therapist prompts for SUDS scores, titrating the intervention to maximise exposure, minimise overwhelming symptoms, and enable habituation as indicated via the child's report and from observation. At the end of every session the child is debriefed and encouraged to practise his relaxation skills and participate in a fun activity with the therapist, to enable him to leave in a more relaxed state.

In vivo exposure refers to the real-life confrontation of traumatic cues or reminders. This is achieved concurrently, usually with the parents'/caregivers' involvement, through application of the techniques learned in therapy to real-life symptoms (e.g., nightmares, triggered emotional responses), via out-of-session activities.

Phase Four: Special Issues and Completion of Therapy

Traumatised and abused children often present with a range of issues. It is likely that many of these will have been addressed throughout the therapy programme; however, this phase enables more specific intervention on residual issues which continue to affect the child or have come to the attention of his parents/caregivers or teacher. Such issues may include anger, guilt and shame, separation, grief and loss, self-esteem and social skills. The STAR Plan is applied to these issues and the child is helped to identify his thoughts and feelings about each issue and to develop strategies for dealing with these responses. During this phase, the therapist may wish to incorporate material from other relevant resources for working with young people – for example, anger management programmes and social skills training.

Completion of therapy is an important process which must be handled with care, including attention to relapse prevention. The fact that therapy is coming to an end can be difficult for some young clients. Children may begin to talk about more symptoms or suffer setbacks during the final weeks of therapy. To help with this phase, the therapist should begin to talk to the child about the end of therapy and acknowledge progress made by the child. She should provide ample support for the child in the belief that he is now ready to do well without her. There should be discussion about possible upcoming difficult situations and how the child might handle them. The child should be encouraged to remember his strengths and social supports as well as his coping skills. In the last session, the child receives a certificate of completion and final reward for participating in the programme and is presented with his scrapbook, which records his therapy progress, to keep.

The therapist should discuss with the parents/caregivers how to support the child in what he has learned and arrange a follow-up phone call or 'booster' session as required.

Use of the TF-CBT programme and limitations

It is expected that therapists will have a suitable level of training in CBT and therapeutic work with child trauma and abuse as a foundation for using this book.

The TF-CBT approach is described session by session. Sessions are designed to take about an hour, although it is recommended that 1½–2 hours are allowed for the exposure sessions (Phase 3), as a longer time frame may be required to allow traumatic events to be processed. The session format is consistent throughout. Each session begins with a statement of overall purpose, followed by the specific goals and materials required. The sessions begin with a review and agenda-setting; activities follow, and the session ends with out-of-session task-setting and a wind-down activity.

The step-by-step approach is designed as a guiding template for applying the treatment strategies. It is anticipated that clinicians will use the programme in a flexible manner, taking account of the individual needs and concerns of each child. Pacing, emphasis and selection of treatment elements will naturally require a degree of skill and experience in working with children and trauma. Therapists are provided with a choice of activities to cater for different developmental needs. The treatment sessions and phases may be flexibly applied to meet individual needs: some children may require self-soothing skills at the outset of therapy; children of cultures with a collective world view are likely to respond to tasks focused on family rather than self in the first session; some children will manage fewer or more activities than those presented for each session; the extent and the depth of the trauma suffered by some children may require further sessions of trauma processing; other children may not require the special issues sessions. Therefore, while designed in a sequence that appears to suit many children, it is intended that session activities and phases will be selected and tailored by therapists to suit the individual child.

There is currently no empirical evidence regarding the optimal length of treatment for traumatised children. Most of the empirically evaluated CBT interventions for childhood mental health disorders have comprised between eight and 16 sessions. Children who have experienced prolonged abuse, premorbid and/or comorbid conditions, or exhibit chronic PTSD with dissociative features, may require longer interventions. Given that PTSD may be a chronic waxing and waning condition in children, judgement based on clinical improvement of symptoms and success in achieving appropriate developmental expectations should determine if and when a child requires further sessions (Cohen *et al.* 2000).

It is important to stress that CBT is no panacea. Some children may not respond to the semi-structured approach and/or the cognitive elements of the programme, or their circumstances may mitigate against complete treatment success. Clinical experience has identified some general prognostic factors. A few children who fall into the age group for which this treatment is designed may not demonstrate the level of cognitive or emotional development needed to manage all elements of the programme. These children may require an initial treatment intervention that is specifically designed to provide replacement experiences to help build more age-appropriate functioning, such as are provided by a neurodevelopmental approach (Perry 2006) or play therapy (e.g., Kaduson 2006).

Furthermore, as for any treatment, for this CBT programme to be truly effective the child must be in a safe environment. Where there are ongoing safety issues the child will invariably fail to maintain treatment gains. Where there are ongoing issues regarding placement, such as uncertainty about whether or not a child will be returning to the care of a parent, the child may minimise past trauma in order not to jeopardise a possible return home. In these cases, the care and protection issues must be addressed and resolved as a priority. If this is happening alongside the therapy, it may be possible to continue the programme and address these issues as part of the therapy. The parent/caregiver sessions can provide a forum to resolve issues that are affecting the child's progress in therapy. This then frees the child to focus on his own healing process in his individual sessions.

A final word on the limitations of any treatment with children: as they are still developing, it is unlikely that all problems will be resolved at once. It is to be expected that some children will require further therapeutic input as they reach new developmental stages or face new situations.

Therapist focus

To summarise the themes presented throughout this introduction: effective and sensitive use of this TF-CBT programme with an individual child and family requires the therapist to maintain a *triple focus*:

1. developing the therapeutic relationship, inspiring hope and participation

2. alleviating symptoms and enhancing coping strategies

3. healing underlying causes of presenting problems.

The phase-based approach is specifically designed to support the therapist in these endeavours: *Phase 1* provides a framework and activities for therapeutic engagement; *Phase 2* provides activities for alleviating symptoms and building coping skills; *Phases 3 and 4* offer processes for healing underlying causes of problems. Of course, all three foci need to be maintained throughout therapy, although typically emphasised in a sequential fashion.

It is important for the triple focus to be employed in conjunction with an ever evolving formulation of the child's presentation and need for therapy. On a session-by-session basis, working with the immediacy of the activities provides here-and-now salient opportunities to distinguish and evaluate the child's responses to situations. In this way, the therapist and child can collaboratively assess the child's progress. For some children, therapy may be complete once they have sufficient sense of control over their symptoms.

For those with more complex problems and ongoing trauma-related symptoms, a shift in therapeutic focus and technique is required. In the context of a trusting therapeutic relationship and with a tool kit of coping skills, this deeper work focuses on underlying causes, such as unhelpful 'meanings' attached by the child to past events, and unbidden responses, such as flashbacks or bad dreams. In *Phase 3*, the therapeutic activities are designed to help the child to face traumatic memories and associated responses and learn to tolerate and emotionally process his traumatic experiences. In this way, the child discovers that these events can be safely left in the past, opening up the possibility of a new view on the present and future.

Phase 4 provides activities designed to further elucidate the 'meanings' (thoughts, assumptions, beliefs) associated with traumatic events in order to help the child (and family) to differentiate their views that are based on fact from those that are misinterpretations of reality, e.g., 'I'm a bad person because I did not protect my sister.' Using the activities, the therapist can assist the child to challenge the old, unhelpful views and begin to develop new more helpful views of self, others and the world. Elucidating and challenging misinterpretations or misapprehensions can often be the turning point in a child's healing. For example, a child who believed that she needed to be with her mother at all times to keep her safe was constantly hypervigilant and on edge, until a session was arranged in which her mother reassured her that she did not need her to keep her safe; that she had other adults to help her with her problems, and that she wanted her daughter to be free of worry and enjoy being a child. Of course, some children's realities are accurate and should be addressed with appropriate interventions – for example, separation and loss with grief work. Behavioural interventions, such as anger management and social skills training, can be used to increase and consolidate new responses. Even so, in stressful situations old responses may re-emerge, which is why relapse prevention is so important and booster sessions are offered.

The overall aim of this TF-CBT approach, as stated previously, is to help the child, over time, to become 'his own therapist', able to effectively manage his thoughts, behaviours, emotions and bodily responses to situations. An added aim is to assist the child and family to lay to rest unhelpful 'meanings' and responses attached to past events, and create new, more helpful responses that can be effectively used in the present and future. These aims are more likely to be achieved by therapists who maintain a triple focus and use case formulation to guide the decision-making process and delivery of the programme elements in an individualised manner.

Assessment

It is expected that prior to embarking on the TF-CBT programme there will have been a comprehensive assessment of the child and his environment in order to establish that this is the most appropriate treatment approach, and to ensure that all elements are in place to enable the best chance of treatment success.

In accordance with child trauma and child abuse literature, the assessment should be multi-modal and multi-informant and comprehensive enough to provide the clinician with a good understanding of the presenting problems as well as predisposing, precipitating and maintaining factors (American Academy of Child and Adolescent Psychiatry 1998; Myers *et al.* 2002; Pearce and Pezzot-Pearce 1994). If screening for diagnostic criteria and co-morbid symptoms is required, a structured interview can be useful, such as the Anxiety Disorders Interview Schedule for Children (Silverman 1987). At the very least, clinical assessment interviews should be conducted with the child, parents/caregivers and significant others, and parent and teacher reports obtained using reliable and valid measures that are acceptable cross-culturally (Achenbach and Rescorla 2007). Child self-report measures useful for children who have experienced trauma and abuse include the Trauma Symptom Checklist for Children (Briere 1996) and the Children's PTSD Reaction Index (Frederick, Pynoos and Nader 1992), or the updated version, the UCLA PTSD Index for DSM-IV (Pynoos *et al.* 1998). For children, both traumatic exposure and traumatic outcomes should be evaluated, as well as resilience and protective factors that can be built on in therapy.

It is important that parents be screened for their own problems, including unresolved trauma or abuse histories, ongoing substance abuse or other mental health problems, interpersonal relationship difficulties, parenting capacity or attachment style that may prevent them from being available to the child in his recovery. Referral for further assessment and appropriate treatment should be made if required.

Clearly, prior to treatment commencing, the child's safety must be ensured and support networks should be in place. In particular, at least one caregiving adult should be able and willing to attend the parent/caregiver sessions and support the child on his therapeutic journey.

Last but not least, it is recommended that clinicians take a scientist-practitioner approach by administering appropriate measures pre-, during and post-treatment in order to assess therapeutic progress and outcome. The fact that this treatment is set out in a step-by-step manner means that it can be used as a basis for research in clinical settings, including by local practitioners using single-case research designs. For monitoring individual responses, and to emphasise the importance of assessing progress, we strongly recommend ongoing evaluation over the course of therapy through use of SUDS or other ratings focused on target problems or goals. Such easy-to-do ratings are not only a gauge of treatment success, they are also a proxy of sorts for treatment fidelity and answering the question 'Is treatment hitting the mark?'

In summary, when embarking on TF-CBT with a child, consider the following:

1. safety of the child

2. parent/caregiver needs and availability to support the child's therapy

3. developmental level of the child and need for replacement experiences

4. the child's attachment relationships and social support

5. cultural considerations

6. presenting problems and treatment priorities

7. tailoring therapy to individual needs and concerns

8. ever-evolving formulation and triple focus

9. pacing, timing and selection of treatment elements

10. ongoing assessment and outcome evaluation.

PHASE 1: PSYCHOSOCIAL STRENGTHENING

PHASE 1
PARENT/CAREGIVER ORIENTATION TO THERAPY

At the completion of the assessment, and before therapy begins, the parents/caregivers[1] are provided with a brief orientation to the TF-CBT programme. This initial orientation may be tagged on to the assessment and carried out with the caregivers and child either together or separately, as judged clinically appropriate.

Purpose

A session to give information to the parents/caregivers about the therapy, encourage their involvement and support, and allow opportunity to discuss questions, concerns and family issues.

SESSION FORMAT
1. Provide information about the therapy

The therapist provides information about the overall goals of therapy, phases of intervention, session frequency and ongoing assessment (e.g., brief assessment of ongoing progress; post-treatment assessment). Additionally, therapists are encouraged to share information about research showing the helpfulness of CBT interventions for child anxiety, PTSD/trauma and abuse-related effects, including the importance of caregiver involvement (Barrett, Dadds and Rapee 1996). Part of the idea here is to instil hope and help develop an expectation of success, as well as to encourage caregiver involvement.

2. Encourage caregiver involvement

The therapist provides examples of how the caregivers can be involved, including a briefing about the self-help tasks that the child will bring home after each session and their role in

---

1   Children may be living with parent(s), extended family or caregivers. The term 'caregivers' will be used to denote the adults who care for the child and are involved with the therapy.

helping the child complete these tasks. This should be linked to a larger discussion about the caregiver role in helping the child learn, consolidate and generalise skills, through active involvement with their child, encouraging, modelling, and reinforcing skill development.

3. Discuss caregivers' questions, child and family issues

The therapist discusses any questions or concerns that the caregivers may have about therapy and any other factors that could affect the child and his ability to benefit from the therapy. The caregivers are encouraged to talk to the therapist about any noticeable changes in the child's behaviour and wellbeing as therapy progresses.

NB If the child is placed with caregivers or living with one parent, but has ongoing access with non-custodial parent(s), it can be useful to involve these parent(s) in the therapy process as well. Of course, these decisions must be made with the child's safety in mind; care must be taken in involving parents in the child's therapy who have been perpetrators of abuse, unless these issues have been addressed and it is clear the child's safety and wellbeing will not be compromised by their involvement in the therapy programme. However, in some cases it becomes evident that the child's ability to benefit from the therapy is limited by issues related to one or both parents and/or other family members. While it is not possible to resolve parental and family issues within the context of this TF-CBT programme, sessions with non-custodial parent(s) and other family members can sometimes be very helpful in assisting the child's therapy progress. For example, a child who is focused on a desire to return to the care of his parent(s) may continue to exhibit trauma symptoms related to the separation until this issue is resolved; in this case, non-caregiving parent(s) may be assisted to tell a child that they are unable to care for him at present, but will always love him and continue to see him regularly. This can free the child to focus on his own personal issues in therapy, and referrals for parent problems can be suggested as appropriate.

PHASE 1
SESSION 1: ENGAGEMENT AND ORIENTATION TO THERAPY

Purpose

The main purpose of this session is to develop the therapeutic relationship, provide an orientation to therapy and to instil hope. Additional information gathering and goal-setting is also carried out.

Goals

- Develop therapeutic relationship, instil hope.
- Orientation to therapy, encourage active participation.
- Introduce workbook.
- Begin information gathering.
- Begin to identify goals for therapy.
- Introduce out-of-session activities.

Materials required

- large scrapbook to be used as a workbook, for sticking in worksheets, etc.
- art materials: drawing paper, crayons, felt tips, paints, coloured pencils
- collage materials: glue, glitter, pictures cut out of magazines, etc.
- a range of age-appropriate games and activities
- 'About me' worksheet
- 'What I'd like help with' worksheet
- 'My account' worksheet

- 'Reward chart' worksheet
- stickers – age- and gender-appropriate
- 'Self-help task 1' – out-of-session worksheet (x 2).

SESSION FORMAT

1. Engagement and orientation

(a) Develop relationship and instil hope

As research shows, the relationship developed in therapy is an important vehicle through which the therapeutic work occurs. The main aim of the first session is to help the child feel comfortable and begin to be able to trust in you as the therapist, and so specific tasks are secondary to the work involved in helping this relationship begin to develop. It is important that the therapist acknowledges, listens to and responds to the child's concerns about being in therapy, and how the decision was made. Proceed slowly, because the therapy situation in itself is one that may provoke anxiety (e.g., a fight/flight/freeze or appease response). Initial discussions should be non-threatening, including an orientation to the therapy room and programme and focus on getting to know each other with the aid of the session activities.

If resistance, anger or anxiety is noted, the child can be given time to think about being in therapy, and to talk it over with his caregivers and the therapist. The therapist's position is that she cannot change what has happened to the child, nor does she want to force the child to participate if there are no problems. Instead, the therapist offers herself as someone who might be able to help with some things that are not going as well as the child would like. The therapeutic relationship is the vehicle by which change happens, and the environment provided must be safe, consistent, predictable, helpful and hopeful. Instil hope by letting the child know that other children like him have found this kind of therapy helpful.

(b) Orientation to therapy room and therapy programme

As part of a non-threatening opening, and following initial introductions, the child can be introduced to the setting and to the overall programme. Accordingly, a first activity can be inviting the child to explore the room and see what activities or games are available, including choosing one to play at the end of the session.

A brief overview of the therapy programme is provided, and should start off in a child-friendly manner (e.g., this therapy is designed to help kids have more fun in their lives). The child should also be asked about what he himself knows about coming along to therapy, what he has been told. Following a discussion about the general reasons for the child's involvement, the therapist can introduce herself more fully (e.g., information about her agency and role) and provide some more specific, child-friendly detail about the programme, including the overall purpose of managing feelings of distress. It should also be emphasised that it is a joint effort ('You and I working together to help you learn about some things to help you feel less upset and to have more fun').

(c) Encourage active involvement

From the outset, ensure the child is given ample opportunity and encouragement actively to participate, ask questions and share his point of view. Show interest in the child by asking about things he enjoys doing, school and family events, and encourage the child to talk freely as a basis for later discussions.

The overall aim is to develop a collaborative relationship based on acceptance and trust, and an expectation of the child's active involvement in the therapy. The session activities that follow are designed to help achieve this aim. Research has shown that a child will engage more freely in discussion when involved in activities such as drawing, collage and games. The activities that are presented in this session and throughout the programme are not intended to be slavishly followed, but rather to be used as a vehicle for achieving the therapeutic goals. That said, activities that represent the essential elements of the programme should of course be included (e.g., reward activities and out-of-session tasks). Likewise, the therapist needs to keep in mind that the step-by-step approach is designed to gradually expose the child to the traumatic experiences that need to be processed. In other words, maintain the *triple focus* discussed earlier (see pages 22–23), and keep the discussion to topics that are appropriate for the individual child and phase of therapy.

2. Session activities

(a) Introduce the workbook

Let the child know that there will be various activities in each session that will be worked on together. These activities will be recorded in the workbook. Reinforce the idea that these activities will help him learn how to handle upsetting feelings and feel better.

(b) Getting to know each other

This should be focused on non-threatening discussions designed to assist the development of the therapeutic relationship as well as gather some information. This can include playing a 'personal facts' game (Kendall *et al.* 1992), where therapist and child take turns in giving information about various aspects of their lives (i.e., non-threatening information to help get to know each other), and then play a quiz game on the answers. (It is important that the therapist remembers all the child's facts, to show interest and help build trust.) The child may like to record some of his own personal facts on the 'About me' worksheet to glue into his workbook.

(c) Picture of self

Ask the child to draw a picture of himself in his workbook. (Adolescents may prefer to make a collage of things they like by choosing pictures cut from magazines and gluing them onto the cover of their workbook.) Use the picture as an aid to understanding the child's sense of self, developmental level, etc. When the picture is finished, ask questions which will cue the child into beginning to distinguish thoughts, feelings and actions, e.g., 'What are you doing in your picture?' 'How are you feeling?' 'What are you thinking?'

Encourage free narrative while this activity is being carried out. For example, ask the child to tell you about a recent event that he enjoyed. Emphasise that you're interested in 'what you feel and think in various situations' (i.e., that his perspective is the important one).

(d) Goals for therapy

Ask the child whether he has thought of anything he would like help with in therapy. Together formulate any goal(s) and record them on the 'What I'd like help with' worksheet. This is just a starting point, and even one goal is enough at this stage, as the worksheet can be added to during later sessions. Instil hope that goals can be achieved. If the child has trouble with this activity, together refer back to the assessment data, which documents his current functioning and trauma symptoms. Note that if there are any immediate distressing problems, the therapist should ensure that behavioural interventions are put in place with the child and the caregivers to address these (e.g., quick relaxation interventions for anxiety).

(e) Introduce the 'Reward chart'

Allow the child to choose a sticker as a reward for participating in the session today. Tell him that he can earn a sticker (older adolescents may prefer points) at each session for completing the within-session activities. A second sticker can be earned each week for out-of-session activities (as discussed in the next section below). The stickers earned will be recorded on a worksheet entitled 'My account' and can be exchanged for rewards at various points in the programme. The therapist and child collaboratively begin to develop a reward chart from which the child can pick, using the 'Reward chart' worksheet. This worksheet can be added to in subsequent sessions; the main idea in the first session is that the child has identified and written on the chart at least one reward that he would like to earn. These may be small gifts appropriate for the child's age, or social rewards, such as playing a computer game with the therapist, or going out for a brief excursion. Decide how many points are required to earn rewards. The child glues the 'My account' and 'Reward chart' worksheets in the back of his scrapbook.

3. Out-of-session activity, summary and feedback
(a) Self-help task

To introduce out-of-session activities, tell the child about the 'self-help' tasks that will be given to him each session. Before discussing the first task, explain that these are to help him practise what he is learning in therapy at home, school and elsewhere.

For his first task, give the child a sample 'Self-help task 1' worksheet. The focus here is on a skill that some traumatised children can have difficulty with – 'remembering to pay attention to the positive'. The task itself is simply to write down a time between this session and the next one when he feels good, and to record what is going on around him (i.e., the situation) and inside of him (i.e., feelings, thoughts) during that time. Help the child complete the first worksheet in the session and reward him a bonus point or sticker for completing of this task. Give the child a blank 'Self-help task 1' worksheet to take home. Check when and where he will do his worksheet, how long he thinks it will take, and who may be available to help if he needs it, as research indicates that increased specificity may promote successful task completion. Modelling and practising the task in session can also help the child to understand how to do it. In addition, remind the caregivers of the between-session task, and of their potential facilitative role (based on their relationship with the child and knowing his specific needs).

(b) Summary and feedback

Provide a brief summary of the session. Ask the child if anything was not clear, how he is feeling, what was helpful/unhelpful, and whether he has any questions or comments. If any important new topics are raised, reschedule for next time.

4. Fun activity

Session 1 ends with a fun activity, as agreed at the outset. One of the therapist's key tasks in Session 1 is to ensure that the child has a good time so that he will want to come back to therapy.

PHASE 1
SESSION 2: RELATIONSHIPS

Purpose

To identify the child's family/caregiving context and support networks. To begin to explore how trauma and abuse has affected the child, his family members and others.

Goals

- Review goals of therapy and out-of-session activity (self-help task); reward effort.
- Identify the child's social context and support networks.
- Explore how trauma and abuse has affected the child, his family and others.
- Identify the child's perceived helpers, and any gaps in the child's support network.
- Introduce new self-help task.

Materials required

- child's workbook
- art materials – paper, scissors, crayons, paints, felt tips, etc.
- 'Paper people' worksheet
- stickers – hearts, bandaids, teddy bears, bees or red dots, spiders or black dots, and yellow dots
- a blank 'Self-help task 1' worksheet may be required
- 'Self-help task 2' worksheets (x 2).

SESSION FORMAT

1. Review and update

(a) Review how the child is today/engagement

Check on how the child is. Schedule a fun activity or game to play together at the end of the session.

(b) Check perception and understanding of the previous session

Briefly review the previous session and goals for therapy. Add any new goals to the 'What I'd like help with' worksheet.

(c) Review self-help task

Here, the idea is to discuss the situation that the child identifies as when he felt good during the past week. Even if the child has not done the task, a discussion should ensue about a time when he did feel good, what was happening both externally and internally, particularly focusing on what might have led to this 'feel-good' situation and the pleasurable feelings and thoughts associated with it. Part of the larger message here is to pay attention to what helps and what leads to feeling good *versus* feeling bad. Participation should be reinforced by recording a point or sticker on the child's Reward chart.

NB If the child has not brought back his 'Self-help task 1' worksheet with at least some indication of effort, check whether his living circumstances are conducive to completing the worksheet at home. If not, it can be negotiated that the child will think about and actively do his task during the week, but actually record it on the relevant worksheet at the beginning of each session. Give the child the opportunity to earn his reward point or sticker by completing a 'Self-help task 1' worksheet in session, using a situation that he remembers from the week.

(d) Set agenda

The therapist briefly outlines what will be covered today, and checks whether there is anything the child wants to talk about.

2. Session activities

(a) 'Paper people'

As trauma in children affects their relationships, and for abused children trauma is interpersonal, and often intra-familial, begin to explore the child's relationships with significant others. Introduce the 'Paper people'[1] activity. Paper dolls are cut out, representing people in the child's life, including himself. Encourage the child to include anyone who has hurt or harmed him. Each person is labelled by writing their names at the top of their head. Stickers are used to show how the child feels toward these people:

- *hearts* for people the child likes or loves

---

[1]   Adapted and used with permission from Lowenstein (2000). See also Crisci, Lay and Lowenstein 1997.

- *bandaids* for people who are hurt or sad
- *bees or red dots* for people who feel mad or angry
- *spiders or black dots* for people who feel scared
- *yellow dots* for people who are to blame
- *teddy-bears* for helpers.

The therapist asks the questions from the worksheet as the child works on the activity, and his answers are recorded. Ask if there is anyone he did not include, and if so, what would he say about them, and what stickers would they get? Note if the child seems to have difficulty identifying anger or fear in relation to family members known to have abused or neglected him. Help the child begin to understand that he may have more than one feeling for the same person, e.g., he may love a family member who also frightens him or makes him feel angry. Spend ample time at the end of the activity identifying the people who help the child and the ways in which they help, to ensure that the child is left feeling strengthened, rather than vulnerable.

It is important that the therapist keeps the *triple focus* idea in mind here (see pages 22–23), as the main aim of this activity is engagement and information gathering. While this activity may begin to function as exposure in a safe therapeutic environment, it is not intended to elicit trauma-related material in any depth at this stage in the therapy. As with other activities, the child can come back to 'Paper people' in later sessions and add more information. It is the therapist who needs to keep discussion to an appropriate level for the individual child.

(b) Additional or optional activity: kinetic family drawing

This activity can be useful if the child has suffered abuse within his nuclear family and the therapist wishes to explore family relationships in more depth. Ask the child to draw a picture of his family doing something together. Note who is included/excluded in the picture, the position and size of each family member, and where the child places himself in the picture. The therapist can use the drawing to ask the child further questions about his family relationships, as required to meet therapeutic goals. For example, ask what each family member in the picture (including him) is feeling and doing, and what each might be thinking.

(c) Reward

Give the child a point or a sticker for his 'Reward chart' for his efforts during the therapy session.

3. Out-of-session activity, summary and feedback
(a) Self-help task

This task follows on from 'Self-help task 1' by having the child again record between sessions when he feels good (and not upset). The task this week includes a time when he feels good with another person or other people, and a time when he feels good on his own. This task is designed to build on the theme of relationships, and also to provide the therapist and child with more information to use within the next session. At the beginning of the next meeting he can share the experiences he wants to share with the therapist. As in the first session, modelling and practice are recommended, as is helping the child make 'public statements of commitment' about specifics related to completing the task (i.e., when, where, how, how long he thinks it will take).

(b) Summary and feedback

Ask the child if anything was not clear, how he is feeling, and whether he has any questions or comments. If any new topics are raised, reschedule for next time. As this session may have raised feelings for the child, ensure that he identifies at least one person who can help him if he feels upset during the week. (Refer to people identified as the child's helpers in the 'Paper people' exercise.)

4. Fun activity

End the session with the fun activity chosen at the outset.

PHASE 1
SESSION 3: TIMELINE

Purpose

To explore the child's history, including good and not-so-good things that have happened in the child's life. To provide psychoeducation on how abuse and trauma can affect children. To introduce the 'STAR Plan', a coping model that the child can use to help himself manage his feelings and overcome challenges.

Goals

- Review self-help task; reward effort.
- Explore the child's history, including history of abuse and trauma.
- Normalise the impact of abuse and trauma on children.
- Introduce a coping model: the 'STAR Plan'.
- Introduce new self-help task.

Materials required

- child's workbook
- art materials – paper, scissors, glue, crayons, paints, felt tips, etc.
- 'The TRAP' worksheet
- 'The STAR Plan' diagram
- 'Self-help task 3' worksheet.

SESSION FORMAT

1. Review and update

(a) Review how the child is today/engagement

Check in how the child is. Schedule a fun activity or game to play together at the end of the session.

(b) Check perception and understanding of the previous session

The therapist briefly reviews the previous session.

(c) Review self-help task

Discuss the two situations identified by the child when he felt good during the week. Reinforce the effort that the child has made, as well as his participation (including a reward point for participation). Discussion should focus on the context and internal reactions, including feelings, thoughts and body reactions. Acknowledge the child's feelings and thoughts that he identified in each situation. Help him take note of pleasurable feelings and what might lead to those feelings.

(d) Set agenda

The therapist briefly outlines what will be covered today, and checks whether there is anything the child wants to talk about.

2. Session activities

(a) Timeline

Ask the child to draw a timeline of his life in his workbook, including good things that have happened, as well as not-so-good things. This should be numbered in years from birth to the present. Different methods can be used, including drawing the timeline like a graph with ups and downs, or as a roadmap of a journey with smooth roads, rough roads, hills to climb, rivers to cross, etc.

The main intention of this exercise is to gather information and to begin to deepen the level of engagement and trust between the therapist and the child. Again, the therapist needs to keep in mind that this exercise comprises an early form of exposure, and must be handled with care (i.e., maintain *triple focus*). It is more important at this stage of the therapy to develop the structure of the timeline with a few key reference points, rather than recording all the details of the child's trauma history. If at any time during the activity the child seems anxious or dissociative, use a quick relaxation technique to help him calm down. For example, instruct him to 'freeze frame', i.e., stop and take a deep breath.

When the child has finished his timeline, the therapist shows respect by thanking the child for sharing his story. Comment that there might be some things he may have forgotten or not wanted to put on the timeline today, that can be added in subsequent sessions (i.e., acknowledge possible avoidance). Acknowledge that when we have had sad, scary or upsetting things happen, thinking about those times can sometimes bring these feelings back.

(b) Psychoeducation about the effects of trauma

Initiate a discussion to reassure the child that many people have feelings that come back after something scary, sad or upsetting has happened to them (including people who are looked up to as brave, or labelled heroes), and that the purpose of this therapy programme is to help him learn to recognise and cope with these kinds of feelings and feel better.

The therapist and child explore together how trauma can affect children, using the 'TRAP' acronym,[1] a simple way of explaining PTSD symptoms to children, based on DSM-IV criteria (American Psychiatric Association 2000):

- **T**rauma – bad thing(s) that happen
- **R**emembering (what happened), even when you don't want to
- **A**voiding things that remind you of what happened
- **P**hysical reactions like heart beating fast, shaking, lashing out.

Using an example of an imaginary child who has had something bad happen, brainstorm together the kinds of reactions he or she might have afterwards. The child writes these ideas on 'The TRAP' worksheet. Cue the child into exploring the range of possible posttraumatic stress symptoms. For example, 'What thoughts or pictures might pop into his mind?' 'Do you think it might affect his schoolwork/relationships/activities/sleeping?' 'What kinds of things might happen in his body?'

To begin to instil hope for a positive outcome, the therapist and child think of a story about a real-life or fantasy hero or heroine (preferably a child, like Harry Potter) who has had something bad happen, and feels upset at times, but copes with his or her feelings and overcomes challenges.

(c) Introduce a coping model: 'The STAR Plan'

Give the child 'The STAR Plan' diagram to glue into his workbook. Explain the symbolism involved: that the STAR shows the way for the child to learn to cope with his feelings and overcome challenges. Keep the symbol plainly displayed in the therapy room and use it on all the materials prepared for the programme. The overall aim is to encourage the child to envisage a hopeful future for himself.

---

1   Adapted and used with permission from Lee James, Leah Giarratano, Psycon Pty Ltd and Talomin Books Pty Ltd. See also Giarratano (2004).

- **S**cary feelings?
- **T**hinking bad things?
- **A**ctivities that can help
- **R**ating and rewards.

Some children may prefer a simpler, more active version with concrete examples of each step:

- **S**top! ('Oh no, I'm feeling bad.')
- **T**hink! ('What am I thinking?')
- **A**ct ('What can I do that will help?')
- **R**ewards ('I did OK; I feel better.')

NB Ultimately the child will be given the opportunity to describe the four steps of the STAR Plan in his own words.[2] The procedure itself will become clear through the examples and practice presented in Phase 2 of the therapy programme, 'Coping Skills' (Sessions 4–8).

(d) Reward

Give the child a point or a sticker on his 'Reward chart' for his efforts during the session.

3. Out-of-session activity, summary and feedback
(a) Self-help task

Introduce 'Self-help task 3'. The child should write on the task sheet twice before the next meeting; this time encourage him to write about an upsetting experience during the week, as well as an experience when he felt happy or relaxed.

---

2   Other versions children have come up with, which may be used if preferred, include:
       1. '**S**tink feelings? **T**hinking bad stuff? **A**ctivities and ideas that can help. **R**ating and rewards.'
       2. '**S**top! Feeling bad? Calm down! **T**houghts that will help. **A**ctions that will help. **R**ewards for me!'

(b) Preparation for the next session

Remind the child that the next meeting between his caregivers and the therapist is due, but that this will not replace 'his time' with the therapist. The therapist should reassure the child that she will not share personal information that he has disclosed, but is interested in what his caregivers think about the therapy and how they can be of help. **NB** For some children and caregivers, joint sessions may be appropriate. This should be discussed and negotiated with the caregivers and the child.

(c) Summary and feedback

Ask the child if anything was not clear, how he is feeling, and whether he has any questions or comments. If any new topics are raised, reschedule for next time.

4. Fun activity

End the session with the fun activity chosen at the outset.

PHASE 2
COPING SKILLS

PHASE 2
PARENT/CAREGIVER SESSION

Purpose

A session to provide caregivers with further information about the therapy, and an opportunity to discuss the child's progress. To introduce the coping skills phase and encourage active involvement.

Materials required

- 'The STAR Plan' diagram
- 'Calm-down tricks' – relaxation techniques for young people.

SESSION FORMAT
1. Provide further information about the therapy

To ensure that caregivers understand the overall goals and strategies of the TF-CBT programme, another brief overview should be provided that links to the one in the initial parent/caregiver session, prior to Session 1. This can include filling in any 'gaps' for the caregivers, which might incorporate any of the following:

1. information about the phases of intervention, frequency of sessions and ongoing assessment and rationale for the inclusion of activities

2. information about the research in relation to interventions for anxiety, including PTSD and abuse and trauma-related effects, in children

3. developing expectations of success and encouraging active involvement of caregivers, including with self-help tasks that the child brings home after each session, and their role in helping the child complete these tasks

4. discussion about the caregivers' role in helping the child to learn, consolidate and generalise skills, through their encouragement, modelling, and reinforcing skill development and the child's active coping attempts

5. encouragement to talk to the therapist about any noticeable changes in the child's behaviour and wellbeing as therapy progresses.

2. Discuss specific ways the caregivers can be involved in the therapy from this point forward

Following on from a general reminder and overview of therapy goals, sessions and strategies, the therapist details progress to date and what is yet to come. First, the first three sessions (Phase 1) are briefly reviewed. Then the therapist explains that the next part of the therapy will be based on the 'STAR Plan', a four-step coping skills plan to help the child identify his feelings and thoughts in upsetting situations, and know what to do to help himself feel better. Explain that the child will have activities each week which will help him to understand the link between his feelings, body reactions, thoughts and behaviours, and learn ideas for changing these in positive ways, rather than resorting to negative behaviours. Encourage the caregivers to assist the child to identify his feelings and thoughts at home, and to practise the relaxation skills he will learn in Session 5. (Show the caregivers the 'Calm-down tricks' worksheet.) Share the idea that progress may not be seen immediately; however, caregivers can be reminded to notice and reinforce the child for using new skills and making active attempts to cope. One idea here is that 'For large change to happen, we as the adults can help by noticing and recognising the small changes that tend to come first.'

3. Caregiver questions, concerns, additional input

Questions should be solicited. The caregivers are invited to ask any questions or share any concerns with the therapist in session, or to call the therapist if they think of additional information that may be helpful, or if they have any further questions.

PHASE 2
SESSION 4: FEELINGS

Purpose

To help the child recognise and manage feelings. To normalise a range of feelings.

Goals

- Review self-help task.
- Introduce the first step of the STAR Plan: 'scary feelings?'
- Normalise a range of feelings.
- Provide a coping model.
- Practise new coping skill: recognition and safe expression of feelings.
- Introduce new self-help task.

Materials required

- child's workbook
- pictures cut out of magazines of people showing different feelings, both facial expressions and entire body postures
- art materials; paint in a range of colours, brushes, paper
- 'All my faces' worksheet (younger children) or 'Feelings chart'
- rewards from the child's 'Reward chart'
- 'Self-help task 4' worksheet.

SESSION FORMAT

1. Review and update

(a) Review how the child is today

Check in how the child is. Schedule a fun activity or game to play together at the end of the session.[1]

(b) Check perception and understanding of the previous session

The therapist briefly reviews the previous session.

(c) Review self-help task

Encourage the child to share the experiences he recorded and discuss his feelings, thoughts and actions at the time. In particular, focus on discussing his feelings, noticing the different feelings he had in each situation. Record a reward point or give a sticker for efforts with the self-help task.

(d) Set agenda

The therapist reminds the child about the STAR Plan and explains that today the session will be about the first part of the STAR Plan: 'Scary feelings?' (or, to be more explicit: 'Scared, sad or mad feelings?') Explain that the work to be done today will help the child to know when he is upset, and what to do about it.

2. Session activities

(a) Identifying feelings

This task is designed to help the child to recognise that different feelings are related to different facial expressions, body feelings and body postures. Have ready a few pictures of people expressing a range of different emotions (these can be cut out of magazines). Ask the child to identify what type of feeling each person might be experiencing, using their facial expressions and body postures as clues. It is important to allow the child free reign to come up with his own ideas, and not to try to correct his interpretations. The activities in this session are also designed to provide opportunities for the therapist to gain insight into the child's understanding and ability to recognise and manage feelings, so as to know which areas to target in therapy.

(b) Guessing feelings game

Introduce this activity as a 'guessing feelings game' or 'mime game' where the idea is to guess the feelings the other person is experiencing from their facial expressions and body postures only. Take turns role-playing with the child, acting out different emotions with body postures and facial expressions but no words (i.e., miming). Take turns to guess the feelings expressed.

---

1   Many children enjoy 'Feelings tic tac toe' as a game to play this session. See Lowenstein (1999).

As with the previous activity, the therapist can use this activity to gain more understanding into the child's understanding of and ability to recognise and express emotion. For example, abused traumatised children can sometimes have difficulty distinguishing sad or angry feelings. Use the time also to normalise the experience of feelings with the child. Discuss how all people have a range of feelings, including, at times, feeling happy or excited, and at other times feeling sad, scared, worried or angry, particularly if they have had scary, sad or upsetting things happen to them – but that people can learn to recognise these feelings and cope with them better.

(c) Modelling coping skills

In addition to normalising, modelling is a useful technique to help children learn new skills. The therapist models the new coping skill of recognition and normalising of feelings as a first step in coping, by giving a brief example of an event that happened to her which made her feel upset. Use a non-threatening, everyday example (e.g., losing something; missing a goal in a sports game). Discuss the feelings that you experienced at the time and how you handled the situation. This should include self-talk that normalises the emotion experienced.

(d) Feelings dictionary[2]

Have ready a range of pictures of people, showing different physical responses to emotions, that the child can use to make a 'feelings dictionary'. The child begins to create his own dictionary by selecting pictures showing different feelings and gluing and labelling them in his scrapbook. Allow the child to label the feelings as he sees them and cue him only as necessary.

(e) Feelings faces

To help the child begin to identify and express his own feelings, ask younger children to complete the 'All my faces' worksheet, on which they draw their happy face, sad face, angry face and scared face. Older children and adolescents can identify feelings they often have by colouring in feelings faces on the 'Feelings chart'. Ask the child to tell you about situations that provoke these feelings. Use coping modelling here to assist the child to self-describe and validate the child's own emotional responses.

(f) Additional/optional activity: painting feelings

Some children respond to a less structured approach. This activity is useful for modelling safe expression of feelings. Provide a large piece of paper (the child may cut this into a shape to represent himself). Invite him to choose a colour to represent each of his feelings, and paint each feeling in a shape on the paper. As above, the activity can be used to assist the child to talk about situations that provoke these feelings and validate the child's responses.

---

2   This activity is adapted from Kendall *et al.* 1990 (see also Kendall *et al.* 1992).

(g) The STAR Plan: recognition and safe expression of feelings

Reinforce the idea that recognising, normalising and expressing our 'Scary feelings' in safe ways can help us feel better.

(h) Reward

Give the child a point or a sticker on his 'Reward chart' for his efforts during the session. If the child has earned eight points or stickers to date, allow him to choose a reward from his 'Reward chart'.

3. Out-of-session activity, summary and feedback

(a) Self-help task

Introduce 'Self-help task 4'. This week the child will write about an imagined person who is worried or upset about something, and will record his ideas about what that person might be feeling and thinking in the situation, picking up clues from facial expressions and body language.

Let the caregivers know about the activity and encourage their involvement and assistance with task completion, if appropriate.

(b) Summary and feedback

Ask the child if anything was not clear, how he is feeling, and whether he has any questions or comments. If any new topics are raised, reschedule for next time.

4. Fun activity

End the session with the fun activity chosen at the outset.

PHASE 2
SESSION 5: BODY REACTIONS

Purpose

To help the child recognise body reactions related to trauma and anxiety, and to introduce relaxation and other self-calming techniques.

Goals

- Review self-help task.

- Expand the first step of the STAR Plan to include body reactions.

- Normalise and model coping with body reactions associated with anxiety and trauma.

- Practise new coping skill: recognition of body reactions, 'freeze-framing', relaxation and other self-calming techniques.

- Introduce new self-help task: develop a rating scale.

Materials required

- child's workbook

- puppets (optional)

- 'Calm-down tricks' – relaxation techniques for young people

- 'Body diagram' worksheet (optional)

- art materials – coloured pencils, felts, paints (optional)

- relaxation tape or CD for children (optional)

- books on relaxation for children (optional)

- 'Self-help task 5' worksheet.

SESSION FORMAT

1. Review and update

(a) Review how the child is today

Check in how the child is. Schedule a fun activity or game to play together at the end of the session.

(b) Check perception and understanding of the previous session

Briefly review the previous session.

(c) Review self-help task

Encourage the child to share the story he recorded between sessions and discuss the feelings, thoughts and actions he guessed the person might be experiencing. In particular, ask the child to describe any body reactions that the person might have experienced. Reward a sticker or point for effort in the self-help task.

(d) Set agenda

The therapist reminds the child about the STAR Plan and explains that today work will continue on the first step of the STAR Plan: 'Scary feelings?' – in particular, feelings associated with body reactions. The session today will help the child to notice his own body reactions and learn ways to calm down when he is feeling upset.

2. Session activities

(a) Identifying body reactions

This activity is designed to help the child begin to identify body reactions linked with feelings and situations. Begin by telling a story about a child excited about something (e.g., a school trip) – and identify together what some of the child's body reactions might be (e.g., jumping up and down, heart beating fast). Then tell a story about several children in an anxiety-provoking situation that is likely to be familiar to the child (e.g., speaking at school assembly, missing the school bus). Ask the child first to describe how they are probably feeling (e.g., anxious, worried, scared), and then to identify what kinds of body reactions these children might experience in this situation (e.g., shaking, sweating, hot face, butterflies in the stomach). Ask the child what body reactions he thinks *he* might experience in both these situations. Also explore how his body feels when he is in a safe situation, to help him begin to distinguish between having a tense body and a relaxed body.

(b) Normalise body reactions associated with anxiety and trauma

Initiate a discussion with the child to normalise the fact that all people have these kinds of feelings in their bodies when they are anxious or worried; and that sometimes these kinds of body reactions come back after people have had something scary, sad or bad happen to them, even when the situation is over. This can include reminding the child about the TRAP exercise from Session 3. The therapist will need to take account of the child's developmental level when wording the following explanation: explain that these feelings are the body's way of preparing us to take action (the fight/flight response), and that they are caused by chemicals (e.g., adrenalin) released when the part of the brain that senses danger (the amygdala) finds a match between the memory of a previous experience and something in the here and now. However, the amygdala often reacts when it doesn't need to, and people can learn to recognise these body reactions and take a moment to pause (like pausing a DVD) and calm themselves down so they can cope better with the situation. This technique is called 'freeze-framing'.

(c) Modelling coping skills and role-play

The therapist describes a situation that she is familiar with which elicits a mild posttraumatic stress response and can be easily role-played. For example: 'Once I got frightened by a dog, and now when I see a dog I have some body reactions.' First, model recognition of body reactions: 'I was at the park and a dog ran towards me…oh, there's that funny feeling in my stomach again.' Then set up a role-play[1] situation with the child – some children may be more comfortable role-playing the situation using puppets. Both the therapist and the child imagine they are in the situation. The therapist describes her emotional and bodily responses, and asks the child to describe his – are they the same or different? Be clear with the child that people can have different reactions to the same situation. The therapist ends the story on a positive note by explaining to the child how recognising her body reactions enables her to 'freeze-frame', take a few deep breaths and calm down, recognise that she is in no immediate danger, and decide to walk on slowly past the dog, rather than run away in fear.

(d) Introduce and practise relaxation and other self-calming techniques

Discuss the idea that when someone is feeling worried or upset it is likely that some parts of their body are also tense. Introduce the idea of relaxation as a way of calming oneself down. (Some children may prefer to use the term 'calm-down tricks' or 'self-soothing' rather than 'relaxation'.) To reinforce the idea that people can calm themselves down using relaxation and other self-calming techniques, practise together the exercises from the 'Calm-down tricks' worksheet: muscle relaxation, deep breathing and imagining a calm scene. Note that children can have quite different preferences for calming themselves down, so it is important for the therapist to be aware of a range of relaxing and soothing techniques and to assess quickly which ones the child responds to best. It can be helpful to ask the child if he has any ways he already uses to calm down, and if so, build on these techniques.

(e) Additional/optional activities

1. Use the 'Body reactions' worksheet, or draw a larger body outline on which the child writes words and/or draws shapes in different colours on body parts to show what

---

1   Note that the role-play procedures used throughout the programme are a form of imaginal exposure. The role-plays can be helpful in that the child may experience anxiety in a safe therapeutic environment, which can facilitate extinction of the anxious response.

happens to his body when he is tense or upset. A second picture can depict his calm, relaxed body.

2. Introduce a relaxation CD for children and practise using it in the session.

3. Read a book on relaxation for children and practise some of the exercises together.

(f) The STAR Plan

Reinforce the idea that when we have 'Scary feelings', our bodies also have those feelings, and that using freeze-framing and calming-down exercises, even just taking a few deep breaths or relaxing tight fists, or doing something already familiar and effective for the child, can help our bodies feel better and give us a chance to stop and think more clearly about our situation.

(g) Reward

Give the child a point or a sticker on his 'Reward chart' for participation during the session.

3. Out-of-session activity, summary and feedback

(a) Self-help task

The self-help task this week combines recognising of body reactions combined with trying some simple self-calming techniques. First, the child is to identify reactions in situations in which he feels worried or upset. A 'Feelings Scale' (SUDS – Subjective Units of Distress Scale) is prepared with the child for recording how strong his feelings and body reactions are to worries and upsetting situations. This should be age-appropriate and drawn with the child on the 'Self-help task 5' worksheet. The range of the scale should be developed by referring to specific experiences identified by the child, from one which could have been worrying, but in which the child was not upset, to one in which he was very upset. The child's range of responses is recorded in his own words. For example, an adolescent might draw a barometer with five or six points on the scale, while a younger child might use a simpler graphic scale with three points (such as faces representing three feeling states in a sequence), as recommended by other treatment programmes (Kendall *et al.* 1992; Kendall *et al.* 1989).

A fairly simple scale might look like this:

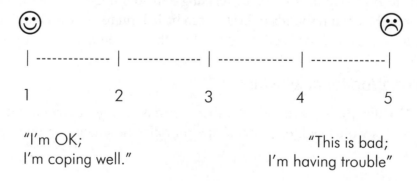

Ask the child to write about an upsetting experience during the week, and to give this a rating with his 'Feelings Scale'. Ask him also to practise relaxation and other self-calming techniques regularly ('practice makes perfect'). Give the child a copy of 'Calm-down tricks' to take home, and any supplementary material (e.g., a relaxation CD if one is available).

Let the caregivers know about the activities, and encourage their involvement and assistance with completing tasks, if appropriate.

(b) Summary and feedback

Ask the child if anything was not clear, how he is feeling, and whether he has any questions or comments. If any new topics are raised, reschedule for next time.

4. Fun activity

End the session with the fun activity chosen at the outset.

PHASE 2
SESSION 6: THOUGHTS

Purpose

To help the child recognise the role of thoughts in both perpetuating and ameliorating symptoms, and learn how to turn anxious or negative self-talk into coping self-talk.

Goals

- Review self-help task.
- Introduce the second step of the STAR Plan: 'Thinking bad things?'
- Provide a coping model.
- Practise new coping skill: recognition of anxious or negative (unhelpful) self-talk; introduce coping (helpful) self-talk.
- Introduce new self-help task.

Materials required

- child's workbook
- 'My experience' diagram
- 'Thought people' worksheet
- pictures of people (preferably children) in anxiety-provoking situations, cut from magazines
- 'Self-help task 6' worksheet.

SESSION FORMAT

1. Review and update

(a) Review how the child is today

Check in how the child is. Schedule a fun activity or game to play together at the end of the session.

(b) Check perception and understanding of the previous session

Briefly review the previous session.

(c) Review self-help task

Review the child's experience with the self-help task, and in particular the relaxation/calming-down exercises. Have the child demonstrate briefly what he did. Discuss how he found recording and rating the upsetting situation, focusing on feelings and body reactions to underline learning from Sessions 4 and 5. If the child mentions any thoughts related to these situations, highlight these as another part of his experience. Reward a sticker or point for effort in the self-help task.

(d) Set agenda

The therapist explains that today the session will be about the second step of the STAR Plan: 'Thinking bad things?' to help the child learn to recognise or 'tune into' his thoughts, and discover that he has some choice about his thoughts or self-talk.

2. Session activities

(a) Recognising the different parts of experience

Reinforce the idea that when things happen, we not only have feelings and body reactions, we also have thoughts and things we do. Show the child the 'My experience'[1] diagram and, using one of the situations described in the child's self-help task, briefly distinguish what might be in each of the shapes. Assist the child to access his thoughts by asking: 'What was running through your mind at the time?' Do not spend too much time on this activity, as the main intention at this stage is to help the child begin to distinguish different aspects of his experiences.

(b) Identifying thoughts

Using the 'Thought people' worksheet, together with the therapist, the child makes up a story about what might be happening for each figure, and fills in possible thoughts (or 'self-talk') in the thought bubbles. This exercise is intended to help the child to begin to distinguish thoughts from feelings, body reactions and actions in different situations.

---

1   Copyright © 1986 Center for Cognitive Therapy, www.MindOverMood.com; adapted and reprinted with permission from Greenberger and Padesky 1995 (p.4).

(c) Recognising self-talk

The therapist helps the child to begin to identify his own thoughts or self-talk by describing an everyday situation and asking him to give examples of thoughts that might run through his mind if this situation happened to him (e.g., you like chocolate ice-cream and there's only vanilla, or your favourite TV programme is on and it's your turn to do the dishes). Ask 'What would be in your thought bubble?' Explore different thoughts that might be possible in the same situation, for example, 'What might someone else think?' This exercise is intended to help the child to begin to recognise his own self-talk, and distinguish different thoughts that are possible in the same situation.

(d) Distinguish helpful thoughts from unhelpful thoughts

Introduce the idea that some thoughts (helpful or 'coping self-talk') may help us cope better with situations, whereas other thoughts (unhelpful or negative thoughts) can make us feel worse and have a negative effect on what we do. For example, if a child misses a goal in a game: 'At least I had a shot at goal; I'll concentrate better next time; I'll do more practice this week,' *versus* 'I'm hopeless; I may as well not try; I should give up this sport.'

The therapist follows this discussion by presenting pictures of real people (preferably children) in anxiety-provoking situations. The child chooses one or two pictures, glues them into his scrapbook and fills in two thought bubbles for each picture, one with unhelpful or negative thoughts that would lead to feeling worse, and the other with thoughts that would help the person cope better with the situation (helpful thoughts). The therapist explains to the child that having more helpful thoughts can help a person feel better.

(e) Coping modelling and role-playing

The therapist reminds the child about the imaginal situation from the previous session (Session 5) in which she coped with a situation that elicited a mild posttraumatic stress response (e.g., having once been frightened by a dog, she is now frightened when she sees a dog running toward her in the park). Using the same example, the therapist describes her initial unhelpful or negative thoughts in this situation, and then explains how she tests these thoughts (e.g., 'The dog is going to jump on me/bite me, etc... But wait, is that really going to happen?'). Ask the child to help think of questions to ask to test the reality of the anxious thoughts. The therapist concludes that she was focusing too much on her anxious or worried thoughts, and by taking a moment to check out the reality of the situation (i.e., using coping self-talk) helps herself calm down and feel better.

(f) Additional/optional activities: recognising and challenging own anxious or negative thoughts; 'thought stopping' and 'thought experiments'

The therapist and child identify the types of situations or events in which the child tends to get anxious or worried thoughts. The technique of 'thought stopping' is introduced: when thoughts seem uncontrollable, say 'STOP' loudly, and immediately think of a more helpful thought. Practise this together, using the previous example. To introduce thought experiments, the child chooses a low-anxiety real-life scenario with which to do a 'thought experiment' together. Ask the child to describe his thoughts in this situation, and, together with the therapist, think of questions to test whether or not his thoughts are realistic. The child and therapist think of some helpful thoughts he could use in this situation. Emphasise to the child that thoughts are ideas, not necessarily the truth. We can believe our thoughts quite strongly and even 'feel' them to be true, but as ideas, thoughts can be tested. Doing 'thought experiments' can help him identify what thoughts he is having about a situation or event, and help him come up with more helpful thoughts. Focusing on these new, helpful thoughts will help him feel better.

NB From this session onwards, the therapist may introduce other cognitive techniques from her own resources, if she considers them therapeutically useful for the individual child. However, for the purpose of this programme (and keeping in mind the need for a *triple focus*) the most important concept for the child to grasp at this stage is the distinction between unhelpful and helpful thoughts.

(g) The STAR Plan

Reinforce the idea that we can recognise when we are 'thinking bad things' and can test such thoughts to check out whether they are realistic in the situation. Anxious, negative or unhelpful thoughts can be replaced with coping or helpful thoughts.

(h) Reward

Give the child a point or a sticker on his 'Reward chart' for his efforts during the session.

3. Out-of-session activity, summary and feedback

(a) Self-help task

The child's self-help task this week is to pay attention to his thoughts or self-talk in situations in which he feels worried or upset. Ask him to write down on the 'Self-help task 6' worksheet his body's reaction and any worried, scared, angry or upset feelings, as well as any unhelpful thoughts and any helpful thoughts that he noticed. Ask him also to practise his self-calming exercises and write down his experiences.

Let the caregivers know about the activities and encourage their involvement and assistance with completing tasks, if appropriate.

(b) Summary and feedback

Ask the child if anything was not clear, how he is feeling, and whether he has any questions or comments. If any new topics are raised, reschedule for next time.

4. Fun activity

End the session with the fun activity chosen at the outset.

PHASE 2
SESSION 7: ACTIVE COPING AND PROBLEM-SOLVING

Purpose

To consolidate active coping with feelings and thoughts. To introduce and practise problem-solving skills. To develop these strategies into steps the child can use to cope with upsetting situations.

Goals

- Review self-help task.
- Review the first two steps of the STAR Plan.
- Introduce the third step of the STAR Plan: 'Activities that can help'.
- Provide a coping model.
- Practise new coping skill: problem-solving.
- Introduce new self-help task.

Materials required

- child's workbook
- white paper, felt tips, crayons, or whiteboard and markers (optional)
- coloured paper or card in at least four different colours
- 'Self-help task 7' worksheet.

SESSION FORMAT

1. Review and update

(a) Review how the child is today

Check in how the child is. Schedule a fun activity or game to play together at the end of the session.

(b) Check perception and understanding of the previous session

Briefly review the previous session.

(c) Review self-help task

In going over the task worksheet, discuss with the child the situations he wrote down during the week in which he felt worried, scared, angry or upset, focusing on how he knew he was upset and his feelings and thoughts at the time. Review the child's relaxation/calming down practice and provide assistance as required to ensure that he is beginning to gain mastery. Reward a point or sticker for efforts with the self-help task.

(d) Set agenda

The therapist reminds the child about the STAR Plan and explains that today the session will be about the third step of the STAR Plan: 'Activities that can help'. Today the child will learn some steps to take to feel better in anxious or upsetting situations, using some ideas learned already, and some new ones.

2. Session activities

(a) Review active coping with feelings and self-talk

Review with the child the two coping strategies already introduced: 'Scary feelings?' (recognising when he is feeling upset, and using self-calming strategies) and 'Thinking bad things?' (recognising unhelpful thoughts, and using more helpful thoughts or coping self-talk). Explain to the child that these are the first two steps of the four-step STAR Plan, which he can use to help himself cope better with upsetting situations.

Encourage the child to develop his own version of the first two steps of the STAR Plan, based on what he has learned so far. Write these steps on cards, using headings such as 'Scary feelings?' for the first, and 'thinking bad things?' for the second. (Use different coloured card to help make the steps distinctive.) The child writes on the first card ideas that he can use to help his feelings and body calm down, and on the second card ideas to help him with his thinking. These steps are explained below in a general way, but should be described in the child's own language.

1. **Step 1**: 'Scary feelings?' – 'Am I feeling worried, upset? I know I can calm down if I try. Use my calm-down tricks – breathing; relax tense muscles, think of a calm scene; remember, feeling nervous is normal.' Explain to the child that by taking Step 1 he will feel calmer and be able to tune into his thoughts, which is Step 2.

2. **Step 2**: 'Thinking bad things?' – stop! 'What are my thoughts/self-talk?' 'I'm worried about…' or 'I'm scared…will happen.' 'Are these helpful thoughts?' 'How else can I think about it?' Explain to the child that Step 2 gives him a chance to stop and notice his thoughts and question whether they are helpful in the situation. If not, what are more helpful thoughts or coping self-talk?

NB The therapist (maintaining a *triple focus* and keeping interventions at a level appropriate for this stage of therapy) should notice any opportunity to begin to access the child's more fundamental thoughts, including 'assumptions' (e.g., 'I must...', 'I have to...', 'I should be able to...') and 'core beliefs' (e.g., 'I'm bad', 'I'm unlovable'). These can be gently challenged as they arise, using Socratic techniques such as asking questions, empathic listening and summarising. For example, *child*: 'I won't be able to cope'; *therapist*: 'How come you think you won't be able to cope?' *Child*: 'There's nobody to help me.' *Therapist*: 'There's nobody to help you?' *Child*: 'Nobody cares about me.' Thought-testing questions can help the child to evaluate these beliefs. (The therapist should adopt a gentle, curious stance, so that the child doesn't experience the Socratic dialogue as an inquisition.) 'What's the evidence?' 'What's an alternative explanation?' 'How does this thought help/not help you (i.e., what are the advantages/disadvantages of this belief)?' These techniques can be used throughout the remainder of the programme, as appropriate for the individual child.

Once the child has written down his own ideas for each of these two steps on the cards, he can glue them into his workbook to refer to later.

(b) Introduce third coping strategy: developing a plan of action ('problem-solving')

Explain to the child that in addition to the first two steps, it can be helpful to do something different to change the situation. This is the third step of the STAR Plan, 'Activities that can help'.

3. **Step 3**: 'Activities that can help'. Make an action plan for solving problems:

- brainstorm ideas for changing the situation: 'What can I do to make this less upsetting?'

- work out which idea has the most chance of success: 'What is the best thing to do?'

(c) Coping modelling and role-playing

Practise problem-solving with an everyday example relevant to the child, such as 'You are about to go to school but can't find your schoolbag. What should you do?' The therapist models the use of brainstorming and encourages the child to think of ideas and suggest which might be the best option. This activity can be made more memorable by actively role-playing the process together. The therapist emphasises that the child will need to practise this skill to get really good at it.

(d) Practise new coping skill: 'problem-solving'

Practise problem-solving with a real-life situation identified by the child. The therapist helps the child to brainstorm alternative actions he could take in the situation and consider which might be the best solution. The main point to make is that by changing what he does (i.e., his actions or behaviour), he will also change the way he feels. For example, a child's problem might be getting annoyed with a younger sibling; by moving away from the situation and going outside to kick a ball around, the child will calm down and feel better.

(e) The STAR Plan

Explain to the child that the skill he has just learned is the third step in the STAR Plan for coping with upset feelings. Help the child to come up with some ideas about things he can do when he is feeling upset, and write these on a card to glue into his workbook. This list can be added to in subsequent sessions. Ideas other young people have come up with include: 'Talk to someone', 'Go to my room and listen to music', 'Write in my diary', 'Go outside and kick a ball'. The child glues the card into his workbook with the other two cards, for easy access.

(f) Reward

Give the child a point or a sticker on his 'Reward chart' for his efforts during the session.

3. Out-of-session activity, summary and feedback
(a) Self-help task

The child's self-help task this week is to begin to use his new skills step by step to cope with situations in which he feels worried or upset, and to record his experiences with one of these situations. Remind the child to use his 'calm-down tricks' as a first step. Give him the 'Self-help Task 7' worksheet to take home.

Let the caregivers know about the activities and encourage their involvement and assistance with completing tasks, if appropriate.

(b) Summary and feedback

Ask the child if anything was not clear, how he is feeling, and whether he has any questions or comments. If any new topics are raised, reschedule for next time.

4. Fun activity

End the session with the fun activity chosen at the outset.

PHASE 2
SESSION 8: RATING AND REWARDS

Purpose

To introduce self-rating and reward as strategies the child can use to cope with perceived failure and acknowledge successful coping. To review and formalise the four-step STAR Plan for the child to use in stressful situations. To prepare the child for the trauma processing phase.

Goals

- Review self-help task.
- Introduce the fourth step of the STAR Plan: 'Rating and rewards'.
- Provide a coping model.
- Practise new coping skill: self-rating and self-reward.
- Introduce new self-help task.

Materials required

- child's workbook
- 'My experience' diagram
- relaxation resources; cassette recorder and tapes (optional)
- 'The STAR Plan' worksheet
- 'Self-help task 8' worksheet.

SESSION FORMAT

1. Review and update

(a) Review how the child is today

Check in how the child is. Schedule a fun activity or game to play together at the end of the session.

(b) Check perception and understanding of the previous session

Briefly review the previous session.

(c) Review self-help task

Review the child's experiences with problem-solving around upsetting situations, including the specific situation he recorded. Reinforce progress and remind the child that learning new skills takes practice. Use the 'My experience' diagram to record the different aspects of the situation as the child experienced it. Notice and comment on any self-evaluation that the child may have experienced as a result of applying his coping strategies, and take note whether he gives himself credit appropriately, as well how he perceives less than total success. Give the child a reward point or sticker for effort in the self-help task.

(d) Set agenda

The therapist reminds the child about the STAR Plan and explains that today the session will be about the fourth step of the STAR Plan: '**R**ating and rewards', in which the child will learn ways to rate and reward his activities and efforts.

2. Session activities

(a) Introduce Step 4 of the STAR Plan

Explain to the child that this is the final step in the STAR Plan for coping with worried and upset feelings. Write the phrase '**R**ating and rewards' on a card for the child to glue into his workbook.

(b) Introduce the concepts of reward and punishment

Discuss the concept of reward as something you receive when you have done well. Use an example, such as teaching an animal a trick, or children getting ticks from the teacher on their work at school to help them learn what is expected. Introduce the concept of punishment, using the example of the child at school – the teacher gives crosses for work that is wrong or not done well. Encourage the child to think of other examples, and discuss how people feel after being rewarded or punished.

(c) Introduce the ideas of self-rating and reward

The therapist introduces the idea that we often think of rewards being given by other people, but actually, we can decide whether we are pleased with our own actions and can rate and reward ourselves. In fact, people often rate and reward or punish themselves for their own thoughts and actions, even though they might not recognise that they are doing this. Use an example relevant to the child, for example, 'Imagine a child won a race at the school sports day.' Discuss how this child might rate and reward himself: what feelings and thoughts might he have; what rewards might he gain? Distinguish between tangible rewards from others (e.g., a certificate) and self-rewards (e.g., thinking 'Wow, I did well!' or telling a friend). Of course, not every child can win, and not winning is not a reason for the child to punish himself. Use a second example of a child who is not successful and does not gain a reward (e.g., he enters a race and comes last). Together come up with a list of possible responses a child might give himself in this instance, for example, 'I'm hopeless at sport; I'll never enter another race,' or 'I didn't get a place, but at least I had a go' (i.e., include some negative and some positive self-responses).

(d) Emotional consequences of self-rating and self-reward

Using the example above, discuss how self-rating can lead to different feelings: negative ratings can lead to feeling upset, sad or angry; positive ratings can lead to feeling pleased or happy. Realistic positive ratings can be a form of self-reward. However, it is important that perceived failure can be reframed as 'learning for the next time', 'At least I gave it a go', and 'Well, it wasn't a total failure because…', so that even an initial 'bad feeling' about perceived failure can be evaluated differently, including identifying partial success, and can set the stage for more success in the future.

(e) Modelling coping skills

The therapist demonstrates the new skill by discussing a time when she coped quite well with a stressful or anxiety-provoking situation and used positive self-rating and reward to acknowledge her success. Examples of self-rating could include realistically assessing your performance, telling yourself you did well, sharing your success with a friend or family member, or giving yourself a treat. It should also include modelling initially perceived failure and re-casting that initial perception into reinforcement for effort, partial success, and a learning opportunity for the next time.

(f) Practise new coping skill: 'rating and rewards'

The child practises the new skill by thinking of an anxiety-provoking situation in which he coped quite well. Use this example to normalise the fact that in any situation it is likely that he will do some things well and others not so well. As already introduced, positive self-rating does not mean looking for 100 per cent success, but rather acknowledging what he did well in the circumstances, as well as what he could have done better. Likewise, self-rewards can be for effort and partial success, even when the overall outcome may not have been successful. The idea here is that the child is encouraged to make a realistic appraisal of his efforts and become his own 'coach' and 'champion for success'.

(g) The STAR Plan

Reinforce the idea that following the four-step STAR Plan will help the child to recognise his feelings, body reactions and thoughts, choose activities to help him cope better with situations, and use positive self-rating and rewards to acknowledge progress and continue to improve coping skills. In addition, even if rewards are not offered freely by others, the child can create his own self-rewards in order to help him feel better and cope better with situations that occur in his life, whether past, present or future.

(h) Reward

Give the child a point or a sticker on his 'Reward chart' for his efforts during the session. If eight points have been earned since the last reward, allow the child to choose a reward from his 'Reward chart'.

3. Out-of-session activity, summary and feedback

(a) Self-help task

Give the child the blank 'STAR Plan' worksheet to take home and complete and ask him to explain the acronym to a parent, caregiver or other significant adult, showing the worksheet to them. Ask him to record an upsetting situation on the 'Self-help task 8' worksheet and to practise using the four-step STAR Plan, taking special note of his experiences with self-rating and reward. Specifically ask the child to focus on rating himself for even partial success, his feelings afterward, and what he used to reward himself.

(b) Preparation for the next phase of therapy

The child should also be reminded that the next meeting between his caregivers and the therapist is due, but this will not replace 'his time' with the therapist. The therapist should reassure the child that she will not share personal information he has disclosed, but is interested in what his caregivers think about the therapy programme and how they can be of help, particularly with regard to practising the STAR Plan at home. Remind the child that the next part of the therapy programme will be different, that he will be practising the STAR Plan while doing some activities to help him cope better with some of the things that may still bother him. Let the child know that for the next part of therapy, longer sessions may be required, up to 2 hours, and that this will be organised with his parents/caregivers.

(c) Summary and feedback

Ask the child if anything was not clear, how he is feeling, and whether he has any questions or comments. If any new topics are raised, reschedule for next time.

4. Fun activity

End the session with the fun activity chosen at the outset.

PHASE 3:
TRAUMA PROCESSING

PHASE 3
PARENT/CAREGIVER SESSION

Purpose

A session to review the STAR Plan and coping skills the child has learned, to check about the child generalising coping strategies at home and in other contexts, and to prepare the caregivers for the trauma processing phase. To allow opportunity for discussion of concerns or problems.

SESSION FORMAT

1. Provide further information about the therapy and review progress

The therapist provides a summary of the therapy programme so far and discusses progress to date and what is yet to come. Specifically, the STAR Plan and coping skills the child has learned are reviewed and the caregivers are asked about the child's use of coping strategies at home and in other contexts. Any general questions about the programme are invited and answered.

2. Discuss specific ways the caregivers can be involved in the therapy from this point forward

The therapist explains that the next part of the therapy will help the child process traumatic past events. This will involve the child re-creating stories about upsetting things that have happened to him in a safe therapeutic environment so that he can put these events in the past and not be so bothered by them in the present or future. The stories will be told using medias chosen by the child, such as paint, clay, sand trays or puppets. The child will use the STAR Plan to help manage any symptoms that arise during this processing. Discussion with the parents/caregivers should cover the possibility of some increase in behavioural symptoms during this phase, and the fact that this is to be expected, and will improve as the issues are addressed. Reassure the caregivers that the child will not be pushed or coerced into talking, and that the therapy will involve the playing out of what happened in ways in which children often naturally process trauma. Explain that while they may initially be reluctant, most children appreciate the opportunity to tell their trauma stories, and find the experience healing. Encourage the caregivers to assist the child by helping him to use the STAR Plan at home. Negotiate the fact longer sessions may be required for the next phase of therapy, up to 2 hours, and discuss how this will be managed.

3. Caregiver questions, concerns, additional input

Questions should be solicited. The caregivers are invited to ask any questions or share any concerns with the therapist in session, or call the therapist if they think of additional information that may be helpful, or if they have any further questions.

PHASE 3
SESSION 9: INTRODUCTION TO IMAGINAL EXPOSURE

Purpose

To introduce trauma processing and have the child practise telling a story, using an imaginal exposure activity. To facilitate ongoing practice of the four-step coping plan.

Goals

- Review self-help task.
- Review the four-step STAR Plan.
- Introduce trauma processing modalities.
- Introduce 'My World' activity.
- Initiate ongoing self-monitoring and use of the four-step coping plan *in vivo*.

Materials required

- child's workbook
- the child's rating scale from Session 5
- a range of creative media for trauma processing – sand tray with a collection of miniature items, clay, art materials, puppets
- 'Self-help task #' worksheet.

SESSION FORMAT

1. Review and update

(a) Review how the child is today

Check in how the child is. Schedule a fun activity or game to play together at the end of the session.

NB While the exposure sessions follow the format of the previous sessions, some flexibility may be required to allow the child to complete his processing with the creative media. Accordingly, the fun activity or game time may be reduced or dropped from the session. The therapist needs to ensure that the child leaves the therapy room in a calm state, but this may be achieved by other means – for example, relaxation and/or debriefing.

(b) Check perception and understanding of the previous session

Briefly review the previous session.

(c) Review self-help task

Review the intervening days with regard to the child's managing of upsetting situations and how he is coping and rewarding himself. Focus particularly on the child's experiences with recalling the acronym 'STAR'. Emphasise any results or rewards that the child may have experienced as a result of applying his coping strategies. Address any difficulties the child reports in using the four steps. Suggest to him that, with practice, the four steps can become almost automatic and not require as much concentration and 'remembering' as they do in the beginning. Reward the child with a point or sticker for effort on the self-help task.

(d) Set agenda

The therapist introduces the range of creative media available and explains that these can be used to tell a story. The child will have the opportunity today to choose a modality and tell a story called 'My World'.

2. Session activities

(a) Change in focus

Explain to the child that the next few sessions are going to include different activities to those used so far. The focus will still include feelings, thoughts and coping skills, but now he is going to be using the ideas he has learned to help him with some other kinds of problems, including helping him to cope better with situations that have happened in the past that still bother him at times. The therapist explains that the STAR Plan can be used to help the child cope with feeling upset about the past, present or future.

(b) Rationale for trauma processing

The therapist explains that while the STAR Plan will help the child cope with upset feelings, there are ways to help these kinds of feelings lessen and go away; and that while it can be helpful to try not to think too much about what has happened in the past, some thoughts and feelings about things that have happened are still inside and can come out at times – for example, as bad dreams or upset feelings when something triggers a memory. Together with the child, think of times when he has these experiences (i.e., his PTSD symptoms). The therapist then explains that telling the story about what happened can help to sort the memories out, so that they do not get in the way any more. The therapist can use the analogy of trauma memories as a jigsaw puzzle scattered on the floor, with pieces getting underfoot – once the child has looked at each piece and fitted them all together, the puzzle is complete and can be put away. Emphasise that lots of other children have found that telling their story to their therapist has helped them get over the bad memories and feel better. Explain that there are different ways to tell their story, and today will be a chance to have a look at the different ways, and practise telling a story using one of these ways.

(c) Introduce trauma processing modalities

The therapist presents the range of modalities she has available to the child. In addition to verbal or written recounting, the child may be offered the following:

- **sand play**: the child uses miniature figures in a sand tray to create a world, scene or story. The child can retell the story, or parts of the story of the trauma, using the miniatures within the sand tray. Facilitated by the therapist, this enables the child to get in touch with the details of what happened, what he was seeing, hearing, smelling, feeling, and what he was thinking. The child gives his completed sand tray a title and tells the story it depicts. He can be asked about the significance of various figures, and which one he would be if he was in the tray. The therapist should be trained in sand play therapy.

- **clay**: the child uses the clay to form shapes to tell the story of the trauma. An example of directions might be, 'Show with the clay what happened.' The child may use the clay to represent a scene, forming realistic figures and objects as he remembers what happened, or he may use the clay more symbolically. Either way, the therapist uses the activity to cue the child into remembering the details of what happened, what he was seeing, hearing, smelling, feeling, and what he was thinking. The child is invited to do whatever he would like with the clay once he has told his story.

- **art**: the child can be offered the choice of a range of art mediums, including paint, crayons, pastels, collage materials and a range of sizes of paper, etc. An example of directions might be, 'Draw a picture of what happened to you.' Older children may prefer to record their story as a cartoon strip. As above, the therapist uses the activity to cue the child in to remembering the details of what happened, what he was seeing, hearing, smelling, feeling, and what he was thinking at the time.

- **puppets**: puppets have been widely used in working with children who find it difficult to talk directly to the therapist about their trauma or abuse. It is useful to have a range of puppets, so that the child can identify particular puppets to represent himself, the abuser and other key people. The therapist invites the child to tell the story of what happened, using the puppets. Alternatively, there can be a therapist puppet and a child puppet, and any conversation can be directed through these. If trauma processing occurs over time, it is important to keep the same puppets in the therapy room.

(d) 'My World' activity

Once the child has chosen the modality he wishes to work with today, introduce the 'My World' activity. Invite the child to make or draw a world with his chosen medium. (If he chooses puppets, ask him to tell a story about a world using the puppets.) The child may choose to create an imaginative world, or a world representative of his real life – it does not matter which, as the purpose of the exercise is primarily to introduce the child to the process. It is likely, however, that the child will choose themes which relate to his own world. The therapist introduces the mode of exposure therapy by ensuring that all conversation is in the present tense. Ask the child to identify who or what he would be if he were in the world. Ask the child what is happening, what he is seeing, hearing, smelling, feeling, and what he is thinking in the situation.

Remind the child about the Feelings Scale (SUDS scale) that he developed in Session 5, and use this to rate the level of comfort/discomfort he would be feeling if he were in this world. Let him know that this scale will be used in the following sessions to help him and the therapist know how he is feeling, and when he may need to use his coping skills.

(e) Practise relaxation or calming strategies

At the end of the activity a few relaxation or other self-calming activities are practised to cue the child into coping strategies that can be used prior to, during and after exposure therapy. Remind the child to continue practising his calm-down tricks at home.

(f) Record the activity

Record the activity in the child's workbook as appropriate. For example, sand trays and clay work should be photographed, dated and named, and given a title. Paintings may be glued into the scrapbook when dry. A brief story may be written about a puppet show. This enables the child to have a visible record of his work, to help him externalise and process his experiences. This may also be shared later with a parent or caregiver.

(g) Reward

Give the child a point or a sticker on his 'Reward chart' for participation during the session.

3. Out-of-session activity, summary and feedback
(a) Self-help task

From now on the child will be given the 'Self-help task #' worksheet on which to record his out-of-session self-monitoring activities. This will facilitate ongoing practice of his new skills in actual situations. Ask him to write down his most upsetting experience during the week, and to describe how he used the STAR Plan, using the acronym to remind himself about each of the four steps.

The therapist continues to encourage caregivers to provide active support for the child during the trauma processing phase, and for using the STAR Plan and completing self-help tasks.

(b) Summary and feedback

The child is asked if anything was not clear, how he is feeling, and whether he has any questions or comments. If any new topics are raised, reschedule for next time.

4. Fun activity

End the session with the fun activity chosen at the outset, if appropriate.

PHASE 3
SESSIONS 10–13: GRADUAL EXPOSURE

Purpose

To use imaginal exposure to create a trauma narrative, and allow emotional processing of trauma memories, using mediums chosen by the child. To help the child to choose trauma topics to work on from his timeline, with gradual exposure from least to most traumatic memories. To continue practising use of the four-step STAR Plan to manage trauma symptoms.

Goals

- Review self-help tasks.

- Introduce gradual exposure activities via chosen modalities.

- Practise use of the four-step STAR Plan to manage trauma symptoms.

- Facilitate ongoing self-monitoring and use of the STAR Plan *in vivo*.

Materials required

- child's workbook

- the child's timeline from Session 3

- the child's rating scale from Session 5

- 'Things that still bother me' worksheet

- a range of media for trauma processing – sand tray and miniatures, clay, art materials, puppets

- 'Self-help task #' worksheet.

SESSION FORMAT

1. Review and update

(a) Review how the child is today

Check in how the child is. Schedule a fun activity or game to play together at the end of the session.

NB While the exposure sessions follow the format of the previous sessions, some flexibility may be required to allow the child to complete his processing with the creative media. Accordingly, the fun activity or game time may be reduced or dropped from the session. The therapist needs to ensure that the child leaves the therapy room in a calm state, but this may be achieved through other means, for example, relaxation and/or debriefing.

(b) Check perception and understanding of the previous session

Briefly review the previous session.

(c) Review self-help task

Ask the child to describe the upsetting experience he had during the week, and how he coped with the situation. Reward a point or a sticker for participation in the task, i.e., the child has demonstrated use of the four-step coping plan.

(d) Set agenda

The therapist reminds the child about telling a story using the creative media in the therapy room, and that the next few sessions will be used to tell his real-life stories about upsetting things that have happened to him and that still bother him; that telling the stories will help him feel less bothered by these memories.

2. Session activities

(a) Trauma processing via gradual exposure

Remind the child that the story he tells today will be a real-life one about something that has happened to him that still bothers him. Refer to the child's timeline and ask him to make a list of the events or situations which still bother him. The child writes these down on the 'Things that still bother me' worksheet, numbering them from least to most upsetting.

During the exposure sessions, the child will work with each trauma memory in turn, beginning with the least distressing, and moving gradually towards the most distressing. Sessions follow on from one another according to the intensity of the trauma, the number of incidents, and the child's own processing. Some children have experienced one particularly intense traumatic incident which may require several sessions to process, while others have experienced multiple incidents, some of which can be grouped together for processing (for example, 'getting hit' or 'parents fighting'). A child invariably has his trauma experiences framed up in his mind in a particular way, and the therapist's job is to access the child's version of events.

Sometimes children require gentle encouragement to begin trauma processing, but once they have experienced telling their story in the first session or so, they are generally most willing to continue the process with more traumatic memories in later sessions. Exposure treatment provides children with an opportunity for greater self-control and self-determination, so it is important that the child sees himself as collaborating and participating in the experience, rather than seeing exposure as something that is done to him.

(b) Introduce trauma processing modalities

The therapist presents the range of modalities she has available to the child. In addition to written or verbal recounting, the following may be offered:

- **sand play**: the child uses miniature figures in a sand tray to create a world, scene or story. The child can retell the story, or parts of the story of the trauma, using the miniatures within the sand tray. Facilitated by the therapist, this enables the child to get in touch with the details of what happened, what he was seeing, hearing, smelling, feeling, and what he was thinking. The child gives his completed sand tray a title and tells the story it depicts. He can be asked about the significance of various figures, and which one he would be if he was in the tray. The therapist should be trained in sand play therapy.

- **clay**: the child uses the clay to form shapes to tell the story of the trauma. An example of directions might be, 'Show with the clay what happened.' The child may use the clay to represent a scene, forming realistic figures and objects as he remembers what happened, or he may use the clay more symbolically. Either way, the therapist uses the activity to cue the child into remembering the details of what happened, what he was seeing, hearing, smelling, feeling, and what he was thinking. The child is invited to do whatever he would like with the clay once he has told his story.

- **art**: the child can be given the choice of a range of art mediums, including paint, crayons, pastels, collage materials and a range of sizes of paper, etc. An example of directions might be: 'Draw a picture of what happened to you.' Older children may prefer to record their story as a cartoon strip. As described above, the therapist uses the activity to cue the child into remembering the details of what happened, what he was seeing, hearing, smelling, feeling, and what he was thinking at the time.

- **puppets**: puppets have been widely used in working with children who find it difficult to talk directly to the therapist about trauma or abuse. It is useful to have a range of puppets, so that the child can identify particular puppets to represent himself, the abuser and other key people. The therapist invites the child to tell the story of what happened, using the puppets. Alternatively, there can be a therapist and a child puppet, and any conversation can be directed through these. If trauma processing occurs over time, it is important to keep the same puppets in the therapy room.

(c) Imaginal exposure activity

Once the child has chosen the modality he wishes to work with today, invite him to tell, make, draw or show his chosen incident or situation with his chosen medium. The child may choose to tell his story in a realistic or a symbolic way. Ask him to identify himself in his story. Using the present tense, ask him what is happening, what he is seeing, hearing, smelling, feeling, and what he is thinking in the situation. Ask him to show from start to finish all the things that happened, and to identify his feelings and thoughts at different times during the trauma processing. Start with the whole event, and then focus on hot spots. 'What is the worst thing about it/the most painful moment?' Care must be taken that exposure sessions are sufficiently long for desensitisation/habituation to occur, and for emotional processing to be promoted (up to two hours should be allowed); repetitive retelling alone is not enough. Encourage more detail and narrative across sessions. As the full context of each event is elaborated, it is no longer encapsulated in a timeless horror, and the meaning changes.

(d) Monitor exposure

The therapist uses the child's Feelings Scale (SUDS scale) to monitor anxiety and distress throughout the imaginal exposure activity. The therapist observes to the child that although he feels upset and anxious as he tells his story, these feelings lessen as he continues to tell more about the situation that he was afraid of. Help the child to notice that telling the story in a safe place helps him to know that it is no longer happening, and that he can start to relax when he thinks about it. Help him to notice that he becomes more relaxed with each session as he works on the memories that once upset him; that the more he confronts these situations, the less they are associated with anxiety, and the less bad they seem than they did before. If anxiety has not been decreasing, comment that this happens sometimes, and encourage the child to tell the story again, perhaps using a different medium. Throughout exposure, the therapist should make reinforcing comments, such as, 'You're doing fine; stay with the image', 'You've done great; you've been very brave to stick it out, even though you said you were quite scared.'

NB It is important for the therapist to acknowledge that there are some memories that will continue to bring up sad or other feelings for the child (e.g., the loss of a parent). In these instances the therapist needs to distinguish grief from trauma, and help the child with grief processing (see Sessions 14–15: Special Issues).

(e) Ending the imaginal exposure activity

The therapist gives the child the opportunity to end the activity as he wishes. For example, some children re-arrange or bury the objects in the sand tray; clay work may be squashed, paintings painted over. These kinds of activities seem to provide the child with symbolic completion and a sense of mastery over the situation.

(f) Practise coping skills

During the imaginal exposure, the therapist reminds the child to use his coping skills as necessary, to help himself calm down. At the end of the activity, a few relaxation exercises are practised. Remind the child to continue practising his calm-down tricks at home.

(g) Record the activity

Record the activity in the child's workbook as appropriate. For example, sand trays and clay work should be photographed, dated and named, and given a title. Paintings may be glued into the workbook when dry. A brief story may be written about a puppet show. This enables the child to have a visible record of his work, to help him externalise and process his experiences. This may also be shared later with a parent or caregiver.

(h) Terminating the exposure phase

After all the events and situations listed by the child have been worked through via imaginal exposure, the therapist and child should review the progress made during therapy. The therapist should check about the extent to which upset feelings and thoughts about the trauma have decreased, and the degree to which the child engages in any previously avoided situations. Any other problems should be identified, to be addressed in the next phase of treatment.

NB If additional exposure sessions are required to complete trauma processing, these should occur, with any extension to the therapy programme being negotiated with all concerned. The recommendation is to extend therapy in two-session blocks with reviews, to keep a sense of focus.

(i) Reward

Give the child a point or a sticker on his 'Reward chart' for participation during the session.

3. Out-of-session activity, summary and feedback

(a) Self-help task

Give the child a 'Self-help task #' worksheet on which to record his out-of-session self-monitoring activities. This will facilitate ongoing *in vivo* practice of his new skills in actual situations. Ask him to write down his most upsetting experience during the week, including his use of the four-step STAR Plan, using the acronym to remind himself about each of the steps.

(b) Preparation for the next phase of therapy

Remind the child that the next meeting between his caregivers and the therapist is due. The therapist should reassure the child that she will not be sharing personal information he has disclosed, but is interested in what his caregivers think about the therapy, and how they can be of help. Check whether there is anything the child would like the therapist to tell his caregivers about his progress. Ask the child whether he would like to share any of his trauma stories with his parent or caregivers.

(c) Summary and feedback

Ask the child if anything was not clear, how he is feeling, and whether he has any questions or comments. If any new topics are raised, reschedule for next time.

4. Fun activity

End the session with the fun activity chosen at the outset, if appropriate.

PHASE 4
SPECIAL ISSUES
AND CLOSURE

PHASE 4
PARENT/CAREGIVER SESSION

Purpose

A session to review the trauma processing phase of the therapy and to identify any special issues or problems to be addressed before therapy ends. This session may be carried out with the caregiver and child jointly or separately, as considered appropriate by the therapist.

SESSION FORMAT
1. Provide further information about the therapy and review progress

The therapist provides a summary of the therapy programme so far, and discusses progress to date and what is yet to come. Specifically, the child's response to the previous phase is discussed, including any noticeable changes in behaviour and wellbeing following the trauma processing. In addition, the child's use of coping skills at home and at school is reviewed. The therapist acknowledges the child's progress and the caregivers' support.

2. Sharing of the child's trauma narrative

If the child has agreed to share his trauma work with the parents/caregivers, this should occur jointly with the therapist, who ensures that the process is safe and positive for the child. Sharing of trauma stories with significant others in a safe therapeutic environment can assist the child's healing.

3. Discuss specific ways in which the caregivers can be involved in the therapy over the last phase and beyond

Encourage the caregivers to assist the child by helping him to continue to use the STAR Plan at home. Prepare the caregivers for setbacks, reminding them that, while the child has new skills, it will still take practice for these to become second nature, and at times problems can be hard for anyone to cope with. For the final phase of therapy, 'Special Issues', ask the caregivers to identify any ongoing issues or problems regarding which they feel the child would benefit from further help. These might include grief and loss, guilt or shame, anger, personal safety, self-esteem, and social skills. The therapist assists the caregivers with specific strategies for alleviating these concerns or problems, as required. Remind the caregivers that the STAR Plan can be applied to any situation in which the child becomes upset. Let the caregivers know that if more than two sessions are required, this will be negotiated.

4. Caregiver questions, concerns, additional input

Questions should be solicited. The parents/caregivers are invited to ask any questions or share any concerns with the therapist in session, or call the therapist if they think of additional information that may be helpful, or if they have any further questions.

PHASE 4
SESSIONS 14–15: SPECIAL ISSUES

Purpose

To help the child identify, understand and manage any special issues associated with his history of trauma and abuse. To continue to practise the use of the four-step STAR Plan and to prepare for completing therapy.

Goals

- Review self-help tasks.
- Identification of special issues, by the child and significant others.
- Work on special issues, using the four-step coping plan and other resources.
- Prepare for completion of therapy.
- Continue self-monitoring, focusing on special issues.

Materials required

- child's workbook
- 'My experience' diagram
- therapist's own resources, e.g., anger management and social skills training programmes, activities to enhance self-esteem, books for young people about healing from abuse, grief and loss, etc.
- 'Self-help task #' worksheet.

SESSION FORMAT

1. Review and update

(a) Review how the child is today

Check in how the child is. Schedule a fun activity or game to play together at the end of the session.

(b) Check perception and understanding of the previous session

Briefly review the previous session.

(c) Review self-help task

Ask the child to describe an upsetting experience he had during the week, and how he coped with the situation. Focus on special issues. It is possible at this stage in the therapy that the child may begin to report that he has not had any upsetting experiences. This is an opportunity to explore any issues that have been identified by others and not by the child himself — for example, behaviour problems at home or at school. Reward a point or a sticker for participation in the task, i.e., the child has demonstrated use of the four-step coping plan.

(d) Set agenda

The therapist reminds the child that the next couple of sessions will be used to help him with any special issues or problems that he may still be bothered about, or that others, such as his parents, caregivers, teacher, social worker or therapist may have noticed.

2. Session activities

(a) Identify and normalise special issues

The therapist helps the child identify any special issues or problems which still bother him. Include problems identified by others. These may include anger, guilt and shame, separation, grief and loss, personal safety, social skills and self-esteem. Explain that these sorts of problems often happen for people who have had upsetting things happen in their lives. Explain that people can learn ways of helping themselves with these kinds of problems, so that they can feel better about themselves and get along better with others.

(b) Understand and manage special issues

It is quite likely that some of these issues will have been addressed as a result of the self-monitoring tasks; however, this is an opportunity to focus on strategies for understanding and managing particular problems.[1] The following are brief outlines for working with three of the

---

[1]   During this phase of therapy it is expected that the therapist will use existing resources available for working with children with special issues, e.g., anger, self-esteem, social skills, and personal saftey programmes. If appropriate, this may include utilising groups which may be available in the child's own community, such as courses for children who have been exposed to domestic violence.

issues particularly associated with abuse and trauma, using the STAR Plan. The same format may be used for working with other issues.

(i) Anger

- **Scary feelings?** To help the child understand what happens when he is angry, ask him to remember a recent time when he felt angry or irritated. Use the 'My experience' diagram to help him describe the situation, his feelings and body reactions. Use the child's Feelings Scale to rate his angry feelings. Remind the child about his calm-down tricks. Ask him to imagine himself back in the situation, and practise using his relaxation to calm himself down.

- **Thinking bad things?** The child identifies his thoughts at the time, and writes these on the 'My experience' diagram. Help the child understand where the anger comes from. People get angry if they think they have been treated unfairly, hurt unnecessarily, or prevented from getting something they expected. It is not just the hurt that makes people angry, but also that expectations were not met. For example, if a person steps on your foot in the bus, whether or not you feel angry depends on your interpretation of the intent and reasonableness of the person's behaviour. Ask the child to think back to the situation and evaluate his expectations and thoughts at the time. What were his expectations? What else could he have thought?

- **Activities that can help.** The child writes on the diagram what he did in the situation. Ask him to evaluate whether this was helpful in the situation or not. Use problem-solving skills to brainstorm helpful actions – for example, recognising early warning signs (body reactions) and using calm-down tricks, walking away and taking time out to relax and think of a better way to deal with the situation.

- **Rating and rewards.** The therapist helps the child to identify the benefits of learning new ways of managing anger, both to him and others.

(ii) Guilt and shame

- **Scary feelings?** To help the child understand the feelings of guilt or shame, ask him to think of a time when he had these feelings. Ask him to describe the situation, his feelings and body reactions.

- **Thinking bad things?** Ask the child to identify his thoughts about the situation. Help him to understand the feelings of guilt and shame. People feel guilty if they have not lived up to the standards they have set for themselves, or they think they have done something wrong. People feel ashamed if they think that what they or a family member has done means that they are 'no good' or 'bad'. Shame can involve a secret, often a family secret. Discuss with the child situations about which he feels guilt or shame. What does he think he should have done? What should others have done, or not done? Were there any secrets involved? What does he think this means about him?

- **Activities that can help.** Explain to the child that overcoming guilt or shame does not necessarily mean letting himself off the hook if he has done something that is wrong in his eyes. It does mean checking out his actions and taking responsibility for what he did or did not do in the situation. It also means making a realistic assessment based on what he could or could not do at the time, given his age and the circumstances, etc. It is also helpful to weigh up how much of the situation was his responsibility, and how much of it was the responsibility of others. To do this, the child lists all the people and aspects of a situation about which he feels guilty or ashamed. Ask the child to draw a circle for a 'Responsibility Pie' and assign slices in sizes that reflect relative responsibility for each person/aspect. For example, Dad (who hit me), Grandad (who used to beat my dad), alcohol (Dad was drunk at the time), Mum (who didn't protect me), me. The child draws his own slice last, so that he does not prematurely assign too much responsibility to himself.

Encouraging the child to talk about secrets associated with shame will help him to experience the therapist's acceptance, running counter to the anticipated criticism or rejection. An aspect of working with guilt and shame is the need for self-forgiveness. A child can be helped to realise that no-one is perfect; we all make mistakes and many people have awful things happen to them, but these things do not mean we are bad, or that life is one mistake after another. If there is anything a child or young person has done, or not done, which has resulted in hurt or harm to another person, he can be encouraged to make amends; for example, by talking to or writing to the other person, if appropriate, or perhaps by helping someone else by way of reparation.

- **Rating and rewards.** The therapist helps the child to understand that talking about these experiences with a trusted person enables him to reassess his feelings, thoughts and actions in relation to what happened. That there are ways of thinking and things he can do to help himself feel better. That regardless of his history, he can live a great life.

(iii) Separation, grief and loss

- **Scary feelings?** Many abused children experience separation, grief and loss in relation to an attachment figure. It is important not to underestimate the impact of this on a child. Attachment is associated with survival, and if an attachment figure disappears or is threatened, even when this person has been abusive, a child is likely to respond in an automatic and instinctive way with a strong emotional response. This may include intense anxiety, overwhelming sadness and/or aggressive behaviour. In addition, a number of abused children have been separated from other family members, such as siblings, and/ or have had multiple caregivers and changes of school. To help the child understand the feelings associated with separation, grief and loss, ask him about people, places and times he misses. The 'My experience' diagram can be used to help him describe the feelings and body reactions he has when he is missing these. Many times the physical sensations associated with separation and grief will be of concern to a child, and it can be a relief for him to discover that these feelings are about missing someone or something important to him.

- **Thinking bad things?** Work with the child to identify thoughts that run through his mind associated with separation, grief and loss. These may take the form of disbelief, denial or confusion (e.g., a child may say of a chronically abusive and neglectful mother: 'Mum only ever gave us little smacks, and she was a good mum, and she's changed now'), or preoccupation, e.g., obsessional thoughts about a parent, leading to intense feelings such as, 'I can't live without her', or, in the case of a child who has had a role in caring for a parent, 'She needs me with her to keep her out of danger.' Thoughts can also be associated with places and times, such as idealising the past before agencies were involved, even though the child was being abused. Discussions with the child around these kinds of thoughts should include some reality testing. This process may be facilitated by enlisting the help of other adults in the child's life, e.g., family members who may be able to help the child accept the truth, and/or a social worker who may be able to assist with factual information. In all circumstances it is important to acknowledge the child's ambivalent feelings about people in his life and his current situation, and to be respectful of his loyalties.

- **Activities that can help.** Explain to the child that helping himself with his feelings and thoughts to do with the people he misses does not mean he no longer cares about them; that even when we don't live with people, or sometimes even see them very often, we still love them. A child may be helped to express his love and caring for people he misses by making cards, writing letters or drawing pictures for them. In addition, creative media, such as sand play and painting, may be used to assist the child to process grief and loss in a similar way to trauma processing. The important tasks for the therapist to help the child with are: (i) to accept the reality of the loss; (ii) to experience the pain of grief; (iii) to adjust to an environment in which these people are missing; and (iv) to be freed up to reinvest emotional energy in his current and future life.

- **Rating and rewards.** The therapist helps the child to identify the benefits to himself and others of 'putting the past in the past' and making the most of his present and future.

(c) Tapering off therapy and preparing for completion of therapy

Remind the child that this is the last phase of the therapy. Ask him to reflect on progress, checking for distortions and attributions. Attribute to the child the progress that has been made; acknowledge him for the way he is dealing with his problems, using what he has learned. Ask the child how he will deal with setbacks, and emphasise that the skills he has learned can be used to help him with all kinds of problems; that he can become 'his own therapist' by using the STAR Plan in any situation.

NB If additional special issues sessions are required, these should occur, with any extension to the therapy programme being negotiated with all concerned.

(d) Reward

Give the child a point or a sticker on his 'Reward chart' for participation during the session.

NB The child's final reward (a social reward) may require some forward planning – for example, if it is to be a party, who will be invited, what food and drink, etc.; or if it is to be an outing (for example, a walk to the local dairy to buy an ice cream), who will come, how much time is required, etc. This should be carefully planned with the child and any adults involved, as appropriate. The reward may comprise part of the 'goodbye celebration' in the final session.

3. Out-of-session activity, summary and feedback

(a) Self-help task

Give the child the 'Self-help task #' worksheet on which to record his out-of-session self-monitoring activities. This will enable ongoing *in vivo* practice of his new skills in actual situations. He will be asked to notice and record situations in which special issues arise, including his use of the four-step STAR Plan, using the acronym to remind him about each of the steps.

The therapist continues to encourage caregivers to provide active support for the child during the special issues phase, and for using the STAR Plan and completing self-help tasks.

(b) Summary and feedback

Ask the child if anything was not clear, how he is feeling, and whether he has any questions or comments. If any new topics are raised, reschedule for next time.

4. Fun activity

End the session with the fun activity chosen at the outset, if appropriate.

PHASE 4
SESSION 16: RELAPSE PREVENTION AND CLOSURE

Purpose

To review and celebrate the child's progress in therapy, to make plans to help the child maintain and generalise his newly acquired skills (relapse prevention), and to bring closure to the therapeutic relationship.

Post-treatment assessment

If a post-treatment assessment is to be completed, this should be carried out with someone other than the therapist immediately prior to this session.

Goals

- Review self-help task.
- Review the child's progress through therapy.
- Relapse prevention.
- Celebrate the completion of therapy and say goodbye.

Materials required

- child's workbook.
- collage materials – paper, scissors, glue, pictures cut from magazines for a 'past–present–future' activity (optional)
- 'Congratulations certificate' celebrating completion of therapy
- materials required for celebration activity – party food, etc.
- 'My STAR Plan' worksheet

SESSION FORMAT

1. Review and update

(a) Review how the child is today

Check in how the child is; respond to any concerns about therapy ending.

(b) Check perception and understanding of the previous session

Briefly review the previous session.

(c) Review self-help task

Ask the child to describe any special issues he experienced during the week, and how he coped with the situation. Reward a point or a sticker for completing the task and confirm that he can cash in his points on his chosen social reward today.

(d) Set agenda

The therapist reminds the child that today will be an opportunity to review what he learned in therapy, to prepare for setbacks, to celebrate his progress and say goodbye. Ask whether he would like to share all or part of this session with his caregiver.

2. Session activities

(a) Review the child's progress through therapy

The therapist and the child (and the caregiver, if invited by the child) go through the child's workbook together, sharing some of the highlights of the therapy experience. The therapist assists the child to reflect on what he has learned about his problems during therapy and gains he has made.

(b) Relapse prevention

The therapist reminds the child (and caregiver) that when therapy ends he can continue to use the STAR Plan to be 'his own therapist'. Give the child a few of the 'My STAR Plan' worksheets to take home, help him fill out the STAR Plan steps in his own words on one of the worksheets ready to use next time he has trouble coping with a situation. Acknowledge relapse as a possible, but controllable, event. Point out that he has skills, but that at times problems can be hard for anyone to cope with; for example, other people can be mean. Ask the child (and the parent/caregiver) about his weaknesses or vulnerable areas. What might be high-risk situations? What might sabotage him in using his coping skills? Rehearse ways of coping with stressors. Encourage the child to remember his strengths and social supports, as well as his coping skills.

(c) Celebration activities

(i) *'Celebration'* activity – the child records in his workbook his strengths, things he is proud of, achievements in therapy and positive aspects of his life, including social supports.

(ii) Alternative or additional activity: *'past–present–future'* collage – a sheet of paper is divided into three sections, headed at the top 'past', 'present' and 'future'. The child chooses a few pictures (from a range of pictures cut from magazines) to represent each, and glues them onto the paper under each heading. This can be a powerful exercise for crystallising in a nonverbal way progress made by the child.

(d) Presentation of certificate

Present the child with the 'Congratulations certificate' commemorating completion of the therapy programme. Encourage the child to continue to use his new skills, and convey confidence in his ability to apply them successfully. Emphasise that regardless of what has happened in the past, he can live a great life!

(e) Celebration, saying good-bye and arranging follow-up

Celebrate the end of therapy with the agreed activity or social reward. Arrangements should be made with the child and caregiver for follow-up as required. A brief phone call to the caregiver after four weeks is recommended, to check how the child is doing and assess whether a 'booster' phone call or session is necessary.

WORKSHEETS

About me

Things I like to do, games, sports, favourite music, movie, book, TV programme, favourite fantasy character or real-life hero…

👍
....

....

👍
....

....

👍
....

....

👍
....

....

👍
....

....

👍
....

....

✓

What I'd like help with...

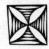 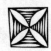

✓ Here is an example you might want to use:
Knowing when I'm upset and knowing what to do about it.

✓
....
....

✓
....
....

✓
....
....

✓
....
....

✓
....
....

My account

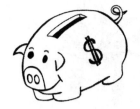

Earn points and redeem for rewards!!

Session #	Date	Points earned

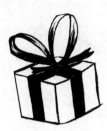

Reward chart

Reward options (items and activities)	Number of points required

Paper people

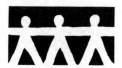

Step 1: Make a string of paper people. Label each person by writing their name at the top of their head. Include yourself, your parents, step-parents, caregivers, brothers and sisters. Include people who have hurt or abused you. Include other people who are important to you, such as relatives, teacher, social worker, therapist, the police, religious leader, close friend, pet.

Step 2: Use the stickers to show how you feel toward these people:

- **Hearts** are for people you **love**. Put heart stickers on the people you like or love.

- **Bandaids** are for **hurt**. Put a bandaid on the people who feel hurt or sad. How come they feel hurt or sad?

- **Yellow dots** are for **blame**. Put dots on the people who are to blame for what happened. Why do you think they are to blame?

- **Bee** stickers or red dots are for **mad**. Put bees on the people who feel mad or angry. Who are they mad at? Why are they mad?·

- **Spider** stickers or black dots are for **scared**. Put spiders on the people who feel scared. Why are they scared?

- **Teddy-bear** stickers are for your **helpers**. Put a teddy-bear on the people who help you. What do they do to help you?

This activity is adapted and used with permission from Liana Lowenstein (Lowenstein, 2000).

✓

The TRAP

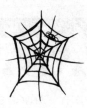

Trauma: What are the bad things that happened?

Remembering: In what ways might bad memories
come back, even when not wanted?

Avoiding: What things might be avoided that are reminders of what happened?

Physical reactions: How do bodies react when feeling scared
or upset because of things that have happened?

The good news is…
The 'STAR Plan' can help you get out of 'The TRAP'…

This activity is adapted and used with permission from Lee James, Leah Giarratano, Psycon Pty Ltd and Talomin Books Pty Ltd. See also Giarratano (2004).

The STAR Plan

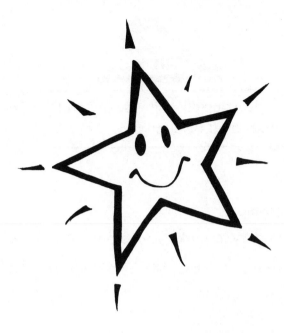

- **S**cary feelings?

- **T**hinking bad things?

- **A**ctivities that can help

- **R**ating and rewards

✓

Calm-down tricks
(Relaxation techniques)

> Exercises you can do to help yourself calm down and feel relaxed when you are becoming anxious, worried, scared or angry:

1. Deep breathing

- Find a comfortable position.
- Take a deep breath and try to make your stomach expand.
- Let out your breath slowly, focusing on how your body feels soft and relaxed as the air comes out.
- Repeat three times.

This is one quick way to help yourself relax when you realise you are becoming anxious or worried.

2. Muscle relaxation

- Make a tight fist by clenching your hand.
- Count to five and focus on how it feels.
- Relax your fist to the count of five and focus on the warm relaxed feeling in your hand.

This can be used when you notice muscle tightness in other parts of your body too, e.g., face, calves – tighten each muscle group to the count of five and relax to the count of five.

3. Imagining a calm scene

- Think of a time or situation in which you were really calm or happy.
- Imagine yourself in that scene and focus on how your body feels.

You can imagine yourself in a calm scene just about any time to help your body feel more relaxed.

4. My own 'calm-down tricks'

- ....
- ....
- ....

All my faces

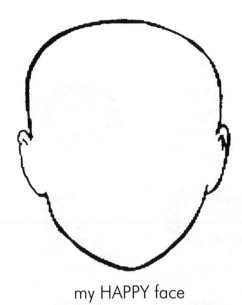

my HAPPY face

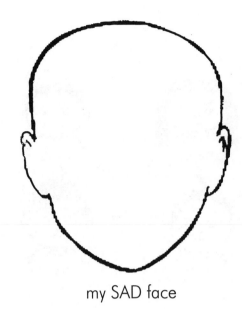

my SAD face

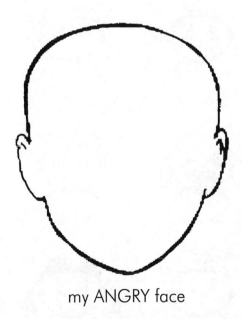

my ANGRY face

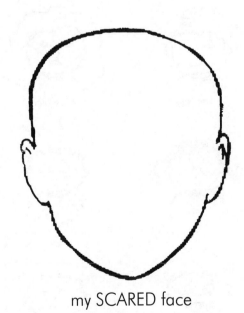

my SCARED face

Feelings chart

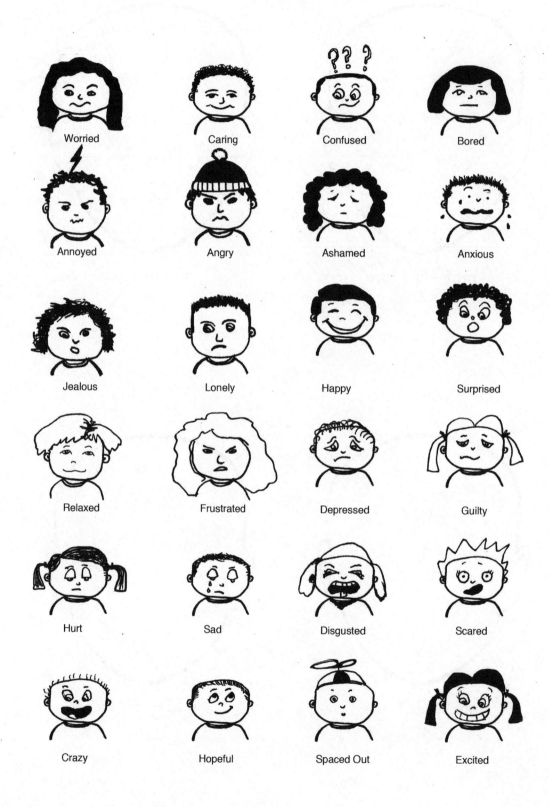

Body diagram

✓

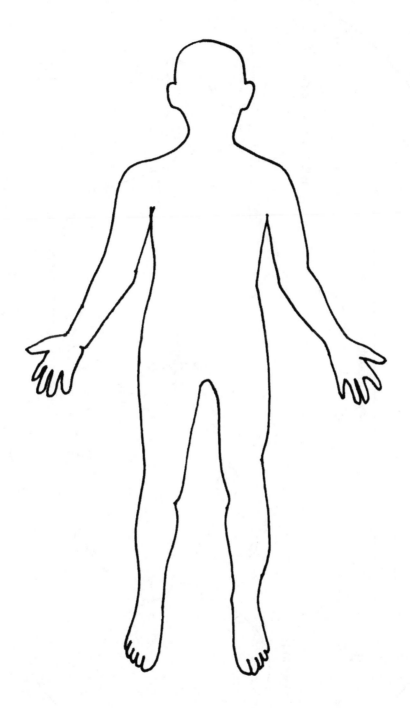

This picture shows what happens in my body when I am:

☐ relaxed and calm
☐ tense or upset

My experience

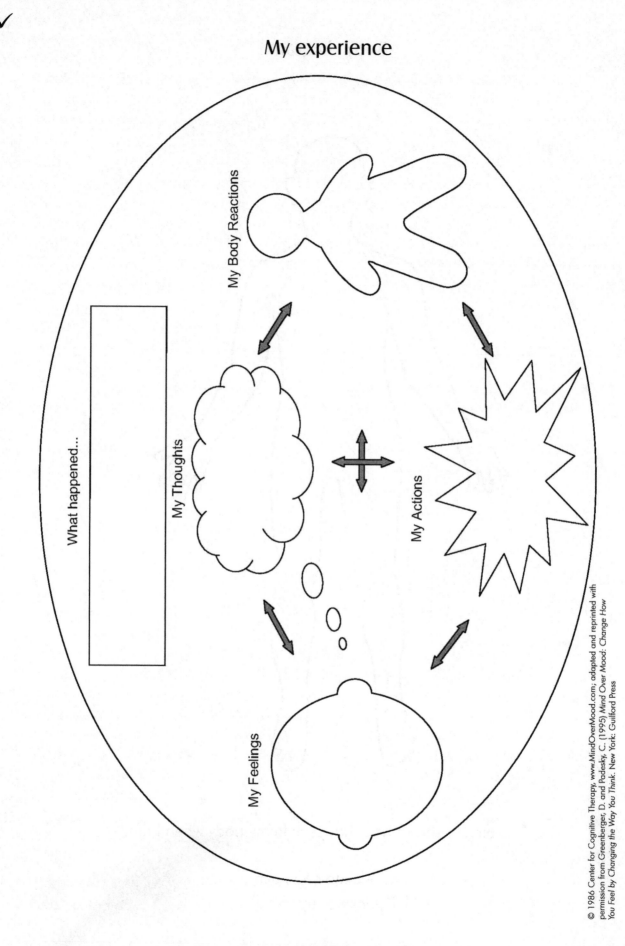

Thought people

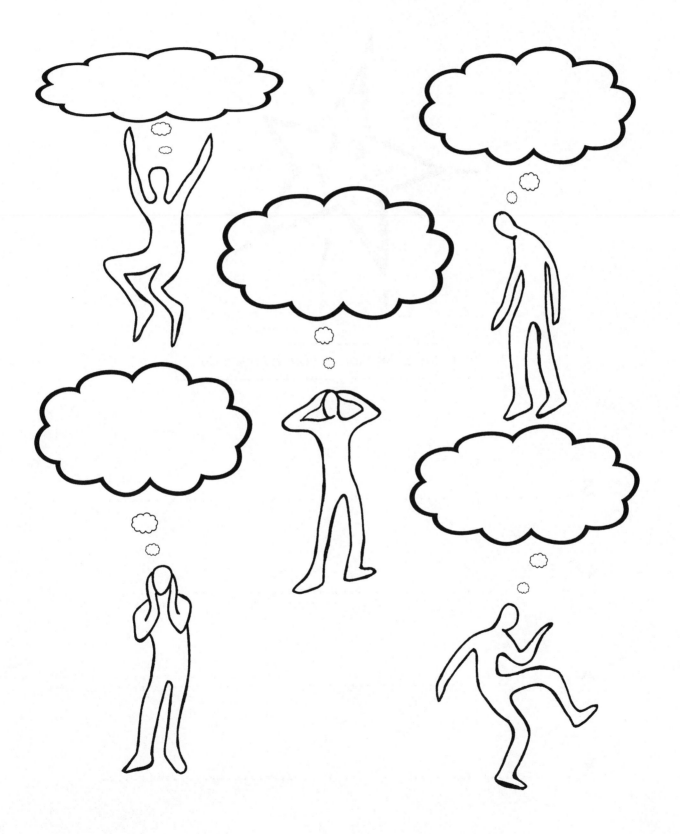

The STAR Plan

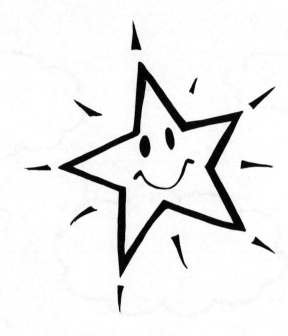

| Fill in the STAR Plan in your own words: |

S ....

T ....

A ....

R ....

Things that still bother me...
(bad memories, things that have happened, bad dreams...)

👎
....

....

👎
....

....

👎
....

....

👎
....

....

👎
....

....

Number these from the least to the most upsetting

✓

Congratulations

This certificate is awarded to:

_____

For excellent participation in The STAR Plan

Signed: _____ Date: _____

Self-help task 1

Name..Date........................

Everyone has good and bad days – we all have times when we feel good, and times when we feel bad. For this week's task, write about a time when you felt really good – like happy or relaxed. What was happening at the time? Did you notice what you were thinking and feeling?.

Time when I felt good:

☺

....

....

....

....

....

....

What was going through my mind when I felt good? What feelings did I notice?

☺

....

....

....

....

....

....

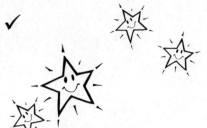

Self-help task 2

Name...Date........................

For this week's task, you're going to write about TWO times when you felt good. First, write about a time when you were with another person or other people, like your friends or family. What was happening? What were your feelings at the time? What were you thinking?

A time this week when I felt good when I was with another person or other people:

😊

. . . .

. . . .

. . . .

. . . .

. . . .

Next, write about a time this week when you felt good when you were on your own. Where were you? What were you feeling and thinking at the time?

A time this week when I felt good when I was on my own:

😊

. . . .

. . . .

. . . .

. . . .

. . . .

Self-help task 3

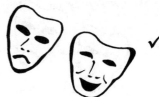

Name...Date...........................

Good job so far! Now that you can write about different kinds of situations, and how you felt, for this week's task you're going to write about a time when you felt good, like happy or relaxed, and another time when you did not feel so good – when you felt a bit worried or upset. Remember – everyone has good days and bad days, and it's OK to have times when you feel upset! Write down what was happening. What were you feeling and thinking at the time?

A time this week when I felt good:

☺

....

....

....

Now, describe a situation this week when you felt a bit worried or upset. What was happening? What were you feeling and thinking? Remember that part of the idea of coming to therapy is to know when you are upset and learn what to do to feel better. You can talk about this situation when you next come to therapy.

A time this week when I felt a bit worried or upset:

☹

....

....

....

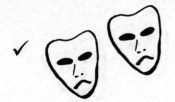

Self-help task 4

Name..Date.........................

> Doing great! This week's task is a little different. Try to IMAGINE someone who is worried or upset. Don't use someone you know in real life – instead, invent a new person. You can give the person any name you want. Now, why is this person upset? What happened? What is the person feeling and thinking?

Make up a situation and write your ideas here:

....

....

....

....

....

Draw a picture to show how this person's face and body might look – if you didn't know the person, what clues would tell us how he or she was feeling?

Clues!

....

Self-help task 5

Name..Date.......................

Now that you've learned some ways to calm yourself down, make sure to practise these calm-down tricks! This week you're going to write about a time when you felt upset, and you tried using your new tricks to calm yourself down. Remember, there are many ways that you can feel 'upset'. Sometimes you might feel worried or scared. Other times you might feel frustrated or angry. You might notice tense or upset feelings in your body as well. Use your 'Feelings Scale' to rate how upset you felt before you used your calm-down tricks, and again after. The idea is to practise all sorts of ways to help yourself feel less upset.

My Feelings Scale:

A time this week when I felt upset

☹ ....

....

....

✓

What I was feeling at the time:

....

....

....

Look at your Feelings Scale. How upset were you, using the scale?

Feelings score: ....

Ways I used to calm myself down

☺ ....

....

....

How did you feel after you calmed yourself down? What was your new feelings score after calming yourself down?

....

....

....

New feelings score: ....

Self-help task 6

Name..Date.........................

> This week write about a time when you felt worried, scared, angry, or upset. Pay close attention to what you were thinking as well as what you were feeling. Remember that sometimes we can think 'helpful' and 'unhelpful' thoughts. Like, when you get a bad mark on a test, a helpful thought would be 'Well, that test was really hard, and I tried my best'. An unhelpful thought might be 'I can't do anything right'. We all have helpful and unhelpful thoughts, at times. This week, when you feel upset, try to notice any unhelpful or helpful thoughts that ran through your mind at the time.

A time this week when I felt upset:

....

....

....

Scary feelings? (my feelings and body reactions at the time)

....

....

....

Thinking bad things? (unhelpful thoughts I noticed at the time)

....

....

....

✓

How I helped myself (what I did to help myself):

☺

....

....

....

Helpful thoughts (helpful thoughts I tried)

....

....

....

Make sure to practise your calm-down tricks! This week when you feel upset, remember to use your tricks to calm yourself down. What calm-down tricks did you use to help yourself this time?

....

....

....

Self-help task 7

Name...Date.........................

> This week write about a time when you felt worried, scared, angry or upset. This time, you're going to pay close attention to activities that can help in this situation, and write these down (these might be activities you tried at the time, or ideas you thought of later). Activities might include an action plan for solving problems, or other things you could do to help yourself in the situation.

A time this week when I felt upset:

....

....

....

STEP 1: Scary feelings? (my feelings and body reactions)

....

....

....

Calm-down tricks I used (how I calmed myself down)

....

....

....

✓

STEP 2: Thinking bad things? (unhelpful thoughts I noticed)

....

....

....

Helpful thoughts (helpful thoughts I used)

☺

....

....

....

STEP 3: Activities that can help (what else I did to help myself in the situation)

☺

....

....

....

Self-help task 8

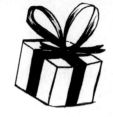

Name..Date......................

Now let's try using self-rating and rewards. During this week write down a time when you felt worried, scared, angry or upset. How did you rate yourself? How did you reward yourself? Did you notice any other good results?

A time this week when I felt upset:

☹

....

....

....

STEP 1: **Scary feelings?** (my feelings and body reactions)

....

....

....

Calm-down tricks I used

☺

....

....

....

STEP 2: **Thinking bad things?** (unhelpful thoughts)

....

....

....

✓
Helpful thoughts

☺

....

....

....

STEP 3: **Activities that can help** (what else I did to help myself)

☺

....

....

....

STEP 4: **Rating and rewards** (how I rated and rewarded myself, even when I tried and it didn't work out like I wanted, and any other good results I noticed)

☺

....

....

....

Self-help task #....

Name...Date........................

> Show how you used the STAR Plan steps to help you cope better with situations.

Situation:

🙁

....

....

....

STEP 1: **Scary feelings?**

....

....

....

Calm-down tricks

🙂

....

....

....

STEP 2: **Thinking bad things?**

🙁

....

....

....

Helpful thoughts

☺

....

....

....

STEP 3: **Activities that can help**

☺

....

....

....

STEP 4: **Rating and rewards**

☺

....

....

....

MY STAR Plan

Name...Date.......................

| Write the STAR Plan in your own words and show how you used it to cope better! |

Situation:

....

....

STEP 1: S..

....

....

STEP 2: T..

....

....

STEP 3: A..

....

....

STEP 4: R..

....

....

RESOURCES FOR THERAPISTS

These resources provide additional material for therapists working with traumatised abused children and their families.

Working cross-culturally

Achenbach, T.M., and Rescorla, L.A. (2007) *Multicultural Understanding of Child and Adolescent Psychopathology: Implications for Mental Health Assessment.* New York: Guilford Press.

Andary, L., Stolk, Y. and Klimidid, S. (2003) *Assessing Mental Health Across Cultures.* Bowen Hills: Australian Academic Press.

Working with child trauma and abuse

Barlow, J. and Schrader, A. (2010) *Safeguarding Children from Emotional Maltreatment.* London: Jessica Kingsley Publishers.

Bentovim, A., Cox, A., Bingley Miller, L. and Pizzey, S. (2009) *Safeguarding Children Living with Trauma and Family Violence.* London: Jessica Kingsley Publishers.

Boyd Webb, N. (ed.) (2006) *Working with Traumatized Youth in Child Welfare.* New York: Guilford Press.

Briere, J. (1992) *Child Abuse Trauma: Theory and Treatment of the Lasting Effects.* Newbury Park, CA: Sage Publications.

Briere, J. and Scott, C. (2006) *Principles of Trauma Therapy: A Guide to Symptoms, Evaluation, and Treatment.* Thousand Oaks, CA: Sage Publications.

Cohen, J.A., Mannarino, A.P., and Deblinger, E. (2006) *Treating Trauma and Traumatic Grief in Children and Adolescents.* New York: Guilford Press.

Giarrantano, L. (2004) *Clinical Skills for Treating Traumatised Adolescents: Evidence Based Treatments for PTSD.* Mascot: Talomin Books.

Gil, E. (2006) *Helping Abused and Traumatized Children: Integrating Directive and Nondirective Approaches.* New York: Guilford Press.

Greenwald, R. (2005) *Child Trauma Handbook: A Guide to Helping Trauma-Exposed Children and Adolescents.* New York: Haworth Press.

Pearce, J.W., and Pezzot-Pearce, T.D. (2007) *Psychotherapy of Abused and Neglected Children* (2nd ed.). New York: Guilford Press.

Perry, B.D., and Szalavitz, M. (2006) *The Boy Who Was Raised as a Dog: What Traumatized Children Can Teach Us About Loss, Love, and Healing.* New York: Basic Books.

Ronan, K.R., and Johnson, D.M. (2005) *Promoting Community Resilience in Disasters: The Role for Schools, Youth, and Families.* New York: Springer.

Sanderson, C. (2009) *Introduction to Counselling Survivors of Interpersonal Trauma.* London: Jessica Kingsley Publishers.

Taylor, J., and Themessl-Huber, M. (eds). (2009) *Safeguarding Children in Primary Care.* London: Jessica Kingsley Publishers.

Cognitive behaviour therapy with children

Deblinger, E., and Heflin, A.H. (1996). *Treating Sexually Abused Children and Their Nonoffending Parents: A Cognitive Behavioral Approach.* Thousand Oaks, CA: Sage Publications.

Friedberg, R.D., and McClure, J.M. (2002) *Clinical Practice of Cognitive Therapy with Children and Adolescents: The Nuts and Bolts.* London: Guilford Press.

Graham, P. (ed.). (2005) *Cognitive Behaviour Therapy for Children and Families* (2nd ed.). Cambridge: Cambridge University Press.

Kendall, P.C. (ed.). (2000) *Child and Adolescent Therapy: Cognitive-Behavioural Approaches.* New York: Guilford Press.

Reinecke, M.A., Dattilio, F.M., and Freeman, A. (eds.) (2003) *Cognitive Therapy with Children and Adolescents: A Casebook for Clinical Practice.* New York: Guilford Press.

Seiler, L. (2008) *Cool Connections with Cognitive Behavioural Therapy.* London: Jessica Kingsley Publishers.

Stallard, P. (2002) *Think Good – Feel Good: A Cognitive Behaviour Therapy Workbook for Children and Young People.* Chichester: John Wiley and Sons.

Working creatively with children

Cattanach, A. (1992) *Play Therapy with Abused Children.* London: Jessica Kingsley Publishers.

Crisci, G., Lay, M., and Lowenstein, L. (1997) *Paper Dolls and Paper Airplanes: Therapeutic Exercises for Sexually Traumatised Children.* Indianapolis, IN: Kidsrights Press.

Labovitz-Boik, B. and Goodwin, E.A. (2000) *Sandplay Therapy: A Step-By-Step Manual for Psychotherapists of Diverse Orientations.* New York: Norton.

Landreth, G.L. (2002) *Play Therapy: The Art of Relationship* (2nd ed.). New York: Brunner-Routledge.

Lowenstein, L. (1999) *Creative Interventions for Troubled Children and Youth.* Toronto: Champion Press.

Lowenstein, L. (2002) *More Creative Interventions for Troubled Children and Youth.* Toronto: Champion Press.

Lowenstein, L. (ed.) (2008) *Assessment and Treatment Activities for Children, Adolescents and Families: Practitioners Share their Most Effective Techniques.* Toronto: Champion Press.

Malchiodi, C.A. (ed.). (2008) *Creative Interventions with Traumatized Children.* New York: Guilford Press.

Whitehouse, E. and Pudney, W. (1996) *A Volcano in My Tummy: Helping Children to Handle Anger.* Gabriola Island: New Society Publishers.

Nicholson, C., Irwin, M. and Nath Dwivedi, K. (eds) (2010) *Children and Adolescents in Trauma - Creative Therapeutic Approaches.* London: Jessica Kingsley Publishers

REFERENCES

Achenbach, T.M. and Rescorla, L.A. (2007) *Multicultural Understanding of Child and Adolescent Psychopathology: Implications for Mental Health Assessment.* New York: Guilford Press.

American Academy of Child and Adolescent Psychiatry (1998) 'Practice parameters for the assessment and treatment of children and adolescents with posttraumatic stress disorder.' *Journal of the American Academy of Child and Adolescent Psychiatry 37,* 4–26.

American Psychiatric Association (2000) *Diagnostic and Statistical Manual of Mental Disorders* (text rev., 4th ed. *(DSM-IV)*). Washington, DC: American Psychiatric Association.

Barrett, P.M., Dadds, M.R. and Rapee, R.M. (1996) 'Family treatment of childhood anxiety: A controlled trial.' *Journal of Consulting and Clinical Psychology 64,* 333–342.

Briere, J. (1992) *Child Abuse Trauma: Theory and Treatment of the Lasting Effects.* Newbury Park, CA: Sage Publications.

Briere, J. (1996) *Trauma Symptom Checklist for Children (TSCC).* Odessa, FL: Psychological Assessment Resources.

Cohen, J.A., Berliner, L. and March, J.S. (2000) 'Treatment of Children and Adolescents.' In E.B. Foa, T.M. Keane and M.J. Friedman (eds) *Effective Treatments for PTSD: Practice Guidelines from the International Society for Traumatic Stress Studies* (pp. 106–138). New York: Guilford Press.

Cohen, J.A., Deblinger, E., Mannarino, A.P. and Steer, R.A. (2004) 'A multi-site, randomised controlled trial for children with sexual abuse-related PTSD symptoms.' *Journal of the American Academy of Child and Adolescent Psychiatry 43,* 393–402.

Cohen, J.A., and Mannarino, A.P. (1996) 'A treatment study for sexually abused preschool children: Initial findings.' *Journal of the American Academy of Child and Adolescent Psychiatry 35,* 42–50.

Compton, S.N., Burns, B.J., Egger, H.L. and Robertson, E. (2002) 'Review of the evidence base for treatment of child psychopathology: Internalising disorders.' *Journal of Consulting and Clinical Psychology 70,* 1240–1266.

Crisci, G., Lay, M. and Lowenstein, L. (1997) *Paper Dolls and Paper Airplanes: Therapeutic Exercises for Sexually Traumatised Children.* Indianapolis, IN: Kidsrights Press.

Davis, L., and Siegel, L.J. (2000) 'Posttraumatic stress disorder in children and adolescents: A review and analysis.' *Clinical Child and Family Psychology Review 3,* 135–154.

Deblinger, E. and Heflin, A.H. (1996) *Treating Sexually Abused Children and Their Nonoffending Parents: A Cognitive Behavioral Approach.* Thousand Oaks, CA: Sage Publications.

Deblinger, E., Stauffer, L.B. and Steer, R.A. (2001) 'Comparative efficacies of supportive and cognitive behavioral group therapies for young children who have been sexually abused and their nonoffending mothers.' *Child Maltreatment 6,* 332–343.

Ehlers, A. and Clark, D.M. (2000) 'A cognitive model of posttraumatic stress disorder.' *Behaviour Research and Therapy 38,* 319–345.

Feather, J.S. (2008) 'Trauma-focused cognitive behavioural therapy for abused children with posttraumatic stress disorder: development and evaluation of a manualised treatment programme.' Unpublished PhD thesis. Massey University, Albany. Available at http://muir.massey.ac.nz/handle/10179/535, accessed 9 April 2010.

Feather, J.S. and Ronan, K.R. (2004) 'Te Ara Whetu: trauma-focused cognitive behavioural therapy for abused children: a treatment manual.' Unpublished manuscript.

Feather, J.S. and Ronan, K.R. (2006) 'Trauma-focused cognitive-behavioural therapy for abused children with postraumatic stress disorder.' *New Zealand Journal of Psychology 35*, 132–145.

Feather, J.S. and Ronan, K.R. (2009a) 'Assessment and Interventions for Child Trauma and Abuse.' In J. Taylor and M. Themessl-Huber (eds) *Safeguarding Children in Primary Health Care.* London: Jessica Kingsley Publishers.

Feather, J.S. and Ronan, K.R. (2009b) 'Trauma-focused CBT with maltreated children: a clinic-based evaluation of a new treatment manual.' *Australian Psychologist 44, 3,* 174–194.

Feather, J.S., Ronan, K.R., Murupaenga, P., Berking, T. and Crellin, K. (no date) 'Trauma-focused cognitive-behavioural therapy for traumatised abused Maori and Samoan children.' Manuscript in preparation.

Finkelhor, D., Ormond, R., Turner, H. and Hamby, S.L. (2005) 'The victimisation of children and youth: A comprehensive national survey.' *Child Maltreatment 10*, 5–25.

Frederick, C.J., Pynoos, R.S. and Nader, K. (1992) 'Reaction Index to Psychic Trauma Form C (Child).' Unpublished manuscript, Los Angeles, CA: UCLA.

Giarratano, L. (2004) *Clinical Skills for Treating Traumatised Adolescents: Evidence Based Treatments for PTSD.* Mascot: Talomin Books.

Greenberger, D. and Padesky, C. (1995) *Mind over Mood: Change How You Feel by Changing the Way You Think.* New York: Guilford Press.

Herman, J.L. (1992) 'Complex PTSD: "A syndrome in survivors of prolonged and repeated trauma."' *Journal of Traumatic Stress 5, 3,* 377–389.

Kaduson, H.G. (2006) 'Release Play Therapy for Children with Posttraumatic Stress Disorder.' In H.G. Kaduson and C.E. Schaefer (eds) *Short-term Play Therapy for Children* (2nd ed.). New York: Guilford Press.

Kendall, P.C., Chansky, T.E., Kane, M.T., Kim, R.S., Kortlander, E., Ronan, K.R. *et al.* (1992) *Anxiety Disorders in Youth: Cognitive-behavioral Interventions.* Needham Heights, MA: Allyn and Bacon.

Kendall, P.C., Kane, M.T., Howard, B.L. and Siqueland, L. (1989) *Cognitive-behavioral Therapy for Anxious Children: Treatment Manual.* Available from Phillip C. Kendall, Department of Psychology, Philadelphia, PA 19122: Temple University.

Kendall, P.C., Kane, M., Howard, B., and Siqueland, L. (1990) *Cognitive-behavioral Treatment of Anxious Children: Treatment Manual.* Available from Phillip C. Kendall, Department of Psychology, Philadelphia, PA 19122: Temple University.

King, N., Tonge, B.J., Mullen, P., Myerson, N., Heyne, D., Rollings, S. *et al.* (2000) 'Treating sexually abused children with posttraumatic stress symptoms: A randomized clinical trial.' *Journal of the American Academy of Child and Adolescent Psychiatry 39*, 1347–1355.

Linning, L.M. and Kearney, C.A. (2004) 'Post-traumatic stress disorder in maltreated youth: A study of diagnostic comorbidity and child factors.' *Journal of Interpersonal Violence 19*, 1087–1101.

Lowenstein, L. (1999) *Creative Interventions for Troubled Children and Youth.* Toronto: Champion Press.

Lowenstein, L. (2000) 'Paper dolls and paper airplanes: Assessing and treating sexually traumatised children.' Workshop presented at the Department of Child, Youth and Family, 24 January, Auckland.

March, J.S., Amaya-Jackson, L., Murray, M.C. and Schulte, A. (1998) 'Cognitive-behavioral psychotherapy for children and adolescents with posttraumatic stress disorder after a single-incident stressor.' *Journal of the American Academy of Child and Adolescent Psychiatry 37*, 585–593.

McFarlane, A.C. and Yehuda, R. (2000) 'Clinical treatment of posttraumatic stress disorder: Conceptual challenges raised by recent research.' *Australian and New Zealand Journal of Psychiatry 34*, 940–953.

Merrick, P.L. (1999) 'The guiding principles of cognitive therapy.' Lecture presented to 75.707 Psychotherapy Theory, Research and Practice. Palmerston North: Massey University.

Murupaenga, P., Feather, J.S. and Berking, T. (2004) 'CBT with children of indigenous and migrant families: Interweaving of cultural context and psychological/therapeutic models with Maori and Pacific Island children and families traumatised by abuse.' Paper presented at the 15th International Congress on Child Abuse and Neglect (ISPCAN), Brisbane, Australia.

Myers, J.E.B., Berliner, L., Briere, J., Hendrix, C.T., Jenny, C. and Reid, T.A. (eds) (2002) *The APSAC Handbook on Child Maltreatment* (2nd ed.). Thousand Oaks, CA: Sage.

National Advisory Committee on Health and Disability (2002). *Improving Maori Health Policy*. Wellington: Ministry of Health.

Nemeroff, C.B. (2004) 'Neurobiological consequences of childhood trauma.' *Journal of Clinical Psychiatry 65*, 18–28.

Pearce, J.W., and Pezzot-Pearce, T.D. (1994) 'Attachment theory and its implications for psychotherapy with maltreated children.' *Child Abuse and Neglect 18*, 425–438.

Perry, B.D. (2006) 'Applying Principles of Neurodevelopment to Clinical Work with Maltreated or Traumatized Children: The Neurosequential Model of Therapeutics.' In N. Boyd Webb (ed.) *Working with Traumatized Youth in Child Welfare*. New York: Guilford Press.

Perry, B.D., Pollard, R.A., Blakely, T.L., Baker, W.L. and Vigilante, D. (1995) 'Childhood trauma, the neurobiology of adaptation, and "use dependent" development of the brain: How "states" become "traits".' *Infant Mental Health Journal 16*, 4, 271–290.

Pynoos, R.S. (1994) 'Traumatic stress and developmental psychopathology in children and adolescents.' In R.S. Pynoos (ed.) *Posttraumatic Stress Disorder: A Clinical Review*. Lutherville, MD: The Sidran Press.

Pynoos, R.S., Rodriguez, N., Steinberg, A., Stuber, M. and Frederick, C. (1998). 'UCLA PTSD Index for DSM-I.' Available from UCLA Trauma Psychiatry Service, 300 Medical Plaza, Los Angelas, CA 90095.

Ronan, K.R., and Deane, F.P. (1998) 'Anxiety Disorders.' In P.J. Graham (ed.) *Cognitive Behaviour Therapy for Children and Families*. Cambridge: Cambridge University Press.

Ronan, K.R. and Johnson, D.M. (2005) *Promoting Community Resilience in Disasters: The Role For Schools, Youth, and Families*. New York: Springer.

Saunders, B.E., Berliner, L. and Hanson, R.F. (2001) *Guidelines for the Psychosocial Treatment of Intrafamilial Child Physical and Sexual Abuse* (Final draft report: 30 July 2001). Charleston, SC: Office for Victims of Crime.

Silverman, W.K. (1987) *Anxiety Disorders Interview for Children*. State University of New York at Albany: Graywind Publications.

Terr, L. (1991) 'Childhood traumas: An outline and review.' *American Journal of Psychology 148*, 1–20.

Yule, W., Smith, P. and Perrin, S. (2005) 'Post-traumatic Stress Disorders.' In P.J. Graham (ed.) *Cognitive Behaviour Therapy for Children and Families* (2nd ed.). Cambridge: Cambridge University Press.